R℞X

Patient Name

Date

Prescription for Life

Richard Furman, MD

Three Simple Strategies to Live Younger Longer

Prescription
for Life

Three Simple Strategies
to Live Younger Longer

Richard Furman, MD, FACS

Я Revell
a division of Baker Publishing Group
Grand Rapids, Michigan

© 2014 by Richard Furman, MD, FACS

Published by Revell
a division of Baker Publishing Group
P.O. Box 6287, Grand Rapids, MI 49516-6287
www.revellbooks.com

Paperback edition published 2015
ISBN 978-0-8007-2444-3

Printed in the United States of America

The Library of Congress has cataloged the previous edition as follows:
Furman, Richard.
    Prescription for life : three simple strategies to live younger longer / Richard Furman, MD, FACS.
        pages cm
    Includes bibliographical references.
    ISBN 978-0-8007-2371-2 (cloth)
    1. Longevity. 2. Self-care, Health 3. Health. I. Title.
    RA776.75.F87 2014
    613.2—dc23   2014015690

This publication is intended to provide helpful and informative material on the subjects addressed. Readers should consult their personal health professionals before adopting any of the suggestions in this book or drawing inferences from it. The author and publisher expressly disclaim responsibility for any adverse effects arising from the use or application of the information contained in this book.

The author is represented by the literary agency of Wolgemuth & Associates, Inc.

15 16 17 18 19 20 21   7 6 5 4 3 2 1

I dedicate this book to those of you who are interested in changing your lifestyle by developing strategies that will lead to a more active, energetic, vivacious existence. Who want to know a medically based strategy to protect your most prized possession: your health. Who realize that much more important than length of your life is the quality of your years.

I dedicate it to you who have the desire to prevent the common health problems that occur with so many as we age: overweight, heart attack, stroke, breast or colon cancer, and, for men, erectile dysfunction. And to you who have had a stent placed in your heart, bypass surgery on your heart, are on a statin drug, or have had a stroke.

It is my desire to inform every one of you how to reach your full physical and mental potential for the rest of your life. I want to teach you how to live longer chronologically, and, even more important, be younger physiologically.

I dedicate this book to you, my reader.

Contents

Foreword: David Jeremiah   11

Preface: Senator Bill Frist   15

Introduction   19

Part 1
What You Need to Understand about the Aging
Process   33

1. Your Course Determines Your Destination   35

2. Your Arteries Are the Cornerstone of the Aging
   Process   39

3. Understanding Cholesterol Is Essential   56

4. Beware of Alternative Ways to Beat Aging   76

5. Prevention Is Key to Staying Young   82

6. Commitment and Action Are Key to Success   90

Contents

Part 2

Eat the Right Foods   115

7. Food Lessons from around the World   117

8. Grocery Shopping Made Easy   124

9. Foods to Avoid   131

10. Foods to Live By   146

11. Off-Limits Foods   159

12. The Effects of Drinking Alcohol   164

Part 3

Reach Your Ideal Weight   169

13. Determining Your Ideal Weight   171

14. The Penalty for Being Overweight   181

15. Weight Loss 101   185

16. Weight Loss Secrets and Easy Steps   195

Part 4

Exercise   207

17. The Most Unrecognized Way to Combat Aging   209

18. The Sedentary Life of a Couch Potato   215

19. Why Exercise Is So Good for You   220

20. The Exercise Plan Everyone Can Follow   228

21. Exercising to Prevent Disease   243

Contents

Part 5

Preventing Dementia   255

22. What Is Good for the Heart Is Good for the Brain   257

Part 6

Preventing Cancer   265

23. The Prescription for Life Plan and Cancer   267

24. The Prescription for Life Plan and Breast Cancer   276

25. The Prescription for Life Plan and Colon Cancer   281

26. The Prescription for Life Plan and Lung Cancer   285

Part 7

Preventing Erectile Dysfunction   289

27. The Causes of Erectile Dysfunction   291

28. What Is Good for Your Heart Is Good for Erectile Dysfunction   297

29. The Prescription for Life Plan and Erectile Dysfunction   301

Conclusion   311

Afterword   313

Prescription for Life 21-Day Plan   319

Medical References   371

Index   384

Foreword

Dr. Richard "Dick" Furman has spent his entire professional life helping people live younger longer. I know because he has helped me! Several years ago, when I was unaware that the lymphoma cancer in my body had recurred, it was my friend Dick Furman who palpated the tiny lymph node hidden underneath a small muscle in my neck. "Tell your doctor to biopsy that node," he said to me. Sure enough, my cancer had returned.

Because he found the malignancy as early as he did, I was able to have it treated before it began to spread. I have been cancer-free now for over twenty years. Dr. Furman's discovery that fateful day was extremely significant, but what he told me later was equally important to me.

He told me that I should make my physical health a higher priority . . . that I should make it my goal to live younger and longer so that I could be used by the Lord for many more years.

His advice changed my life. I realized that I had neglected my body by not exercising regularly. I was also unknowingly eating many of the wrong foods and slowly gaining unwanted weight. I believe God allowed my cancer and my meeting with

Dr. Furman for my ultimate benefit, and that is why I am so excited about this book.

Prescription for Life is the result of hundreds of hours of research, which is evident by the over one-hundred-fifty sources at the end of the book. But this is not just another medical book about the causes of bad health; this is what the title says it is: a prescription for life—a strategic plan to develop the healthiest life and body possible.

Included in the prescription is straightforward advice about the importance of lifestyle change, the significance of attaining an ideal weight, and the necessity of developing a personal exercise routine.

While many respond negatively to the thought of exercising, dieting, and changing their lifestyle, Dr. Furman has managed to take what is threatening and make it thrilling. When you finish this read, you will actually be excited about the possibility of a longer, healthier life.

Recently, while traveling in Israel, I saw a sign in a Jerusalem store window. I had just finished reading Dr. Furman's book, and the message on this sign grabbed my attention: "We don't stop playing because we are old; we are old because we stop playing." I had been learning a similar lesson: "We don't stop exercising because we are old; we are old because we stop exercising."

Prescription for Life does more than simply diagnose the problems of aging; it presents the exact steps necessary for taking control of your future health. Dr. Furman points out that while many people have a desire to stay as young as possible, very few have the necessary commitment to make any substantial changes in order to achieve their goal.

As you will discover in this book, there is a vast difference between desire and commitment. Desire is of the mind; commitment is of the heart. In these next few pages, you are going to learn how to translate your desire into a plan and determination to make your personal health a priority for the rest of your days on this earth.

I want to encourage you as Dick encouraged me: Stay as vivacious and as physiologically young as possible so you can enjoy an active and productive life. Today, my health is one of my most prized possessions. It ought to be yours as well. What you are about to read is not going to simply suggest that you do something to enhance your health; it is going to demand that you make certain changes in your lifestyle, in the control of your weight, and in the development of a personal exercise program.

At the end of this book, you will discover another important secret about a quality life. I hope you will wait until you have read all of the up-front chapters before you jump to the end. But in case you're wondering . . . here's a hint: C. S. Lewis is reported to have once said that "our bodies and our souls live so close together that they catch each other's diseases."

I will make this promise to you: if you will determine to read and understand what Dr. Furman's medical research substantiates concerning your physical well-being, and if you commit yourself to the plan of action that he suggests in this book, you will give yourself the best opportunity to live younger longer.

Through my experience with cancer, I was faced with my own mortality. It was a very serious and sober time in my life, and I began to realize the precious value of each and every day. But experiencing cancer or having a heart attack is not a necessary requirement for making important changes. Why not let what you read in this book be your wake-up call to a better life.

David Jeremiah

Preface

Have you ever wished you had a friend who was a doctor? Someone who could explain in straightforward terms what is happening to you as you count the days to another birthday?

Consider the book you hold a letter from a friend who can do just that. Dr. Dick Furman can be that friend to you—as he is to me—and I appreciate what he has done by writing a book everyone can understand and apply.

I know Dick and his motivation behind this book. When you spend days with someone in a thatched-roof mud hut and perform surgery in a makeshift operating room with only flashlights to illuminate the operative site, you get to know someone pretty well. Those are memories Dick and I made during our yearly trips to mission hospitals throughout Africa when I served in the United States Senate. I know his heart. He realizes he can save more lives and help more people to live younger with *Prescription for Life* than he did in his productive career as a surgeon operating one-on-one.

My own surgical career consisted of heart and lung transplantation, whereas Dr. Furman specialized in thoracic and vascular surgery. We both realize that the health of your arteries is one of the major factors in aging. In my own professional life as a doctor, I soon realized that most people are not aware of what they can do to fight aging. They simply don't know. But all that changes with this book and this plan.

This book spells out the three most helpful components in extending whatever your life expectancy is today by five to seven years. And Dr. Furman underscores that, in addition to longer life, you can achieve a much higher quality of life, one with more energy and leading to more productivity and fulfillment.

What I like most about what you are about to read is that it is medically factual. So much of what the popular press reports is the latest trend, fad, or the opinion of one. In contrast, what Dr. Furman lays out is the result of a thorough review of the medical literature, written in layman's terms that are easily understood.

What you will read is based on findings reported in the latest peer-reviewed medical literature. The most conclusive research findings are typically based on controlled studies with two groups. For example, in weight-loss studies, one group adopts certain interventions or changes in lifestyle and the other group—similar in all other regards—does not. Then researchers compare outcomes and draw conclusions about the effectiveness of the specific changes in lifestyle.

Using this same principle, Dr. Furman discusses three strategies that will enable you to become physiologically younger: eating the proper foods, exercising, and achieving ideal weight.

Based on my professional observations drawn from caring for thousands of patients over the years, I humbly predict that you will make lifestyle changes as you read this book because of the clarity with which Dr. Furman explains the issues.

Change begins with understanding the "why." This book informs you about specific foods you will want to simply quit eating once you realize they cause blockage in the arteries that feed your heart (leading to a heart attack) and your brain (resulting in a stroke), as well as in the artery that causes erectile dysfunction when it is blocked. You will learn an easy-to-remember foundation of foods you should be eating to be more energetic and actually feel and act younger than your present chronological age. It works, and each recommendation is grounded in current medical knowledge.

You will soon understand why, from a medical sense, it is imperative to move toward and arrive at your ideal weight. As a surgeon, I saw daily the numerous problems associated with being overweight. It even affects two of our most common cancers—colon and breast cancer. (And most women want to do everything possible to prevent breast cancer.) What you are about to read gives you the statistics and facts that support why reaching an ideal weight is preventive as well as therapeutic.

As a heart specialist—having spent most of my career replacing diseased hearts with healthy ones—I want to underscore the section on exercise as it relates to the strength and health of your heart. All other organs of the body depend on your heart for their nutrients and oxygen; it should be your most prized muscle. The stronger your heart muscle mass is, the less work it has to do each time it beats. Remember, your heart is beating in your chest around one hundred thousand times a day! You will learn to determine how effectively your personal pump is functioning, as well as learn a simple routine to make certain it is as strong as possible.

As you read *Prescription for Life*, you will learn how to live in a way that adds another seven to twelve years to your life, and, equally important, you will learn how to live to feel better and more energetic each day. As for me—and I am sure for you as well—I want to stay as young as possible as I get older.

Read it. Apply it. If you do, and you are like the majority of Americans, you will become seven to twelve years younger physiologically than you are chronologically.

You may even feel young enough to want to go and sleep in a thatched-roof mud hut somewhere in the world.

Bill Frist, MD
Senate Majority Leader, U.S. Senate

Introduction

"If only I had known."

Those are the saddest words a doctor can hear from someone who has just been diagnosed with a severe health problem—one that could have been prevented. But you are about to learn how to prevent the most common health problems that damage your body. I know this is a bold promise, but once you have read this book, you will never need to say, "If only . . ."

You *are* going to know. This book will tell you—clearly. What you do about it, however, will be your decision.

I have been a thoracic and vascular surgeon for over thirty years. I've operated on blockages of arteries throughout the body—arteries to the heart, to the brain, to the kidneys and the legs. With my own hands, I have opened arteries that were blocked with so much plaque that vital blood flow was completely choked off. I have bypassed a blockage of plaque by taking veins out of a patient's leg, sewing one end of the vein into an artery in front of a blockage, and sewing the other end into the artery past the blockage. I have opened the main artery leading to the brain and used a miniature spoon to dissect out plaque that was blocking 95 percent of the blood flow to that half of the brain.

More than half of all Americans, as well as people in many other countries with similar lifestyles to ours, will die because of the war going on inside their arteries. I have been fighting this war all my surgical life, cleaning out those blockages. I have come to the realization that doctors who operate on the arteries in the heart, those who place stents and sew in bypasses, do nothing to cure heart disease. Without a change in lifestyle on the part of the patient, the same damage to the arteries continues after the treatment is done.

So instead of operating on the symptoms of aging, I have decided to try to save lives by teaching people how to *prevent* what causes the demise of more than half of Americans. In this book, I want to help you prevent the underlying disease process by teaching how to put a halt to the cause. In fact, I'm going to tell you some secrets for which you might thank me for years to come.

Because of a lifetime of research, I have also learned that a huge part of the process we call aging is strategically preventable. So this book will also open your eyes to the most important facts about the aging process. And I am going to help you, one step at a time, begin to turn back the clock of aging. I will keep it simple and straightforward. And as crazy as this probably sounds, five years from now you will be seven to twelve years younger, physiologically, than your chronological age. You will be more active than the majority of your friends, even if they are many years younger than you.

You will learn a three-part, strategic lifestyle plan that will change you. I will teach you what to eat and how to work on your weight until you reach your ideal number of pounds. If you are already at that weight, I will give you some easy pointers for how to maintain it every day. I will take you down the road, step-by-step. And exercise will become a routine part of your life.

Whatever your life expectancy is today, you are going to extend that number by seven to twelve years. But what is even more important is that the years you have left will be quality years.

I know the aging process is inevitable, but because of what I have learned in a lifetime of experience, I also know that the rate of that process can be controlled and, many times, reversed. And best of all, those extra years you are adding to your life expectancy are going to be active, vivacious, vibrant years that you will enjoy. When you commit to the Prescription for Life plan, you will take control of your physiological aging process rather than simply sit by and watch it happen.

It is my desire to show you how to reach your full potential in your physical and mental performance—for the rest of your life!

My First Week in Medical School

I remember my first day of medical school like it was yesterday. "The heart is the single most important organ in your body," our professor told us in anatomy lab. He went on to compare the heart to the brain, explaining that someone can be comatose—brain dead—but be alive because the heart is still pumping blood throughout the body. That anatomy class was exciting, because I actually got to hold a human heart in my hand. I was able to look closely at the muscle makeup. I could see each artery lying on the surface of the muscle. When the professor spoke of the anterior descending coronary artery, I could see it, touch it.

He then had us gather around the dissecting table to give us a lecture. He had several cadaver hearts laid out on the slab, some with the muscle cut through and some with the arteries spliced open longitudinally to show blockage within the vessels.

He wore a white lab coat, all three buttons neatly through each button hole. His head was freshly shaved, but you could tell he was mostly bald to begin with. And his shoes were shined. His appearance was enough to make you pay attention to what he was about to say, but my eyes were fixed on what he held out toward us in his hands. In each, he had a human heart, both split open, showing directly into the main chamber.

I have never forgotten what he said next: "The heart in my right hand belonged to a gentleman who was what I call a couch potato. He was grossly overweight. Never exercised a day in his life, and from his medical records, we know he was on numerous medications." He laid the heart in his left hand on the dissecting table and pointed to the wall of the couch potato's heart.

"As you can see, the wall of his left ventricle is only millimeters thick. His heart was a poor excuse for a pump he depended on every minute he was alive. Remember the thickness. Autopsy results reveal that he died from a massive heart attack—at the age of fifty-two."

He placed it on the table and picked up the other heart. I looked closely and thought I saw some blood dripping from the opened chamber but quickly realized there was no blood in the organ since the autopsy had been done. (Those were formaldehyde drops.)

"This man's heart is different. You see the thickness is a good three centimeters. It was strong right up to its last beat. His report said he was someone who was trim, who took good care of his body, didn't smoke, and was a frequent tennis player. This heart belonged to a sixty-one-year-old gentleman who died in an automobile accident. He was physiologically younger than the fifty-two-year-old couch potato. If you want to live younger, the only advice I can draw from these hearts is to be as active as you can."

Next he showed us a heart in which he had opened an artery longitudinally. He passed it around. The inside of the artery was as clean as a whistle. Then he passed around several hearts that had partial or complete blockages within the inside of the arteries. He pointed out that most of the cadaver hearts he received from people who had died a non-accidental death had such blockages. He didn't know the actual cause of the blockages, but he knew they were the cause of the heart muscle not getting the oxygen it needed, resulting in the demise of that particular patient.

Then he made another statement I've never forgotten: "The ones with the least amount of blockage are the ones who lived longer."

My first week of medical school amazed me. I could hardly wait to tell my future wife about holding a human heart in my hands. That weekend, I packed my books into the car and took off to see her. I was so excited that I even wanted to take a heart with me to show Harriet all the exciting things I had learned. So I slipped one out of the building as I left, rationalizing that I wanted to study its valves and arteries over the weekend.

Of course, I knew the real reason was to show Harriet what a human heart looked like inside and out. I could hardly wait to get to her house with my surprise floating inside a jar of formalin.

After two and a half hours of traveling and the usual ritual of giving Harriet a hug and kiss, I reached into the car to retrieve my brown paper sack. I removed the jar containing the heart, ready to demonstrate my newly learned knowledge.

Harriet shifted away from me and quickly took three steps backward as I began my lecture. She showed slight interest, but it was evident that I would not be taking the heart out of the jar to show her any of the details. I couldn't believe she didn't have the interest I thought she ought to. If Harriet was to be a doctor's wife, she ought to want to hold a real heart—at least that was the way I looked at it. However, I accepted reality and placed the jar on the driver's seat of my car.

Harriet and I had decided to talk with her parents that evening about moving up our wedding plans. We had intended to wait until I completed my first two years of medical school so I could devote all my time to studying and she could finish college. However, I learned that the medical school would hire med students' wives to work as office assistants, giving us income, and I thought there was no reason to wait so long to marry. After dinner, we sat in the living room with her parents, and I explained that Harriet and I would like their blessing to move ahead with our plans.

Harriet's dad was tall and thin, with curly hair and glasses. He just looked over the top rim of his glasses toward me, not at me but at a spot somewhere between my eyes and the floor. "I've always wanted my daughter to graduate from college," he said. Then he got up from his La-Z-Boy recliner and walked back toward their bedroom.

Harriet's mother smiled and said, "I had better go back with him." At least she smiled.

This was not the response I'd hoped for. All I could do was turn to Harriet and tell her, "When you get back to school Monday, find out what day your class will graduate two years from now, and we will plan to get married the following Saturday."

As I got into my car to drive back to school the next day, still with two years in front of me before our wedding, I picked up the jar holding the heart and placed it on the passenger seat. I looked at it for a moment and thought, *My anatomy professor is correct. Whether it's a cadaver's dead heart in a jar or a live "broken" heart in the human thorax of a disappointed fiancé, the heart is the single most important organ in your body.*

It is still hard for me to understand why Harriet didn't share my excitement over learning about that heart. And today I know even more about hearts than I did then; I know about a lifestyle that can make you younger physiologically, and I want to share that knowledge with others.

Yet, so many seem about as interested in changing their lifestyle as Harriet did in holding a human heart. If you want to live life to the fullest, you need to commit to taking your heart "into your own hands." It will be the most important decision you will ever make about how you live the rest of your life. If you want to better your life, I invite you to read this book to the very end. The story is not over until you learn all three lifestyle strategies and how they are interrelated for your best life.

As I look back on what my anatomy professor taught me years ago and review today's medical literature, it is easy to explain what the professor concluded. While it wasn't known back then, the medical journals today show exactly how much exercise you need to strengthen your heart muscle to be actively younger. The literature reveals the significance of being at an ideal weight. And the same literature tells you exactly what foods cause those blockages in your arteries.

Exercise. Weight. Diet. All three strategies intertwine to prevent those obstructions and allow you to live longer.

LIVING YOUNGER

It doesn't matter what your chronological age may happen to be.
Money can't buy a younger life.
It's not for sale.
But you can have it . . . for free.

Decisive Moments

Hopefully, there comes a time when you realize there are things you can do to improve yourself. Galatians 6:7 in the King James Bible says, "Whatsoever a man soweth, that shall he also reap." Some people realize this truth too late in life in terms of their health. They look back on their years and grasp the terrible truth that they should have sown differently. I am glad I realized this reality earlier in my journey.

I remember the moment well. I was forty-two years old and trying on a new pair of pants during an annual sale. As I tried to button the pants at the waist, I realized they were just too tight. Twice before, I had to buy pants with a bigger waist size, and now I was faced with the same situation. In that moment, I made a decision. I folded the trousers and neatly hung them back on their hanger.

"I will come back later. These just don't seem to fit properly," I said to the salesman as I handed him the pants. What I said to myself was that I would get my weight back to what I remembered as an ideal weight. That happened to be what I weighed when I finished high school. I had stayed at that weight throughout college but only for a few months once I started medical school. I remembered ideally weighing 140 pounds. Even though I stayed in fairly decent shape, I'd slowly added twenty-one pounds, mostly around my waist.

Ideal Weight

After that *moment of decision*, it took about three months to lose my excess weight. My new rule was to eat nothing between meals or after dinner. No snacks. I also would have no desserts and eat smaller portions. When I got to what I had deemed my ideal weight, I went back to the men's shop and bought new pants. I had to pay the regular price, but I knew I would be able to wear those pants until they wore out. I was committed to remain at my ideal weight for the rest of my life. I didn't realize it then, but I had just accomplished one-third of the lifestyle I needed for the rest of my life. The medical literature would teach me the rest of what I needed to learn to keep my body as young, physically and mentally, as possible.

I did not realize that moment of decision would change my future as much as it did. I knew I felt better at my ideal weight and that medically it was the right thing to do. But I didn't realize it was only my first step toward the quality of life I wanted.

Exercise

It wasn't too much later when I read in a medical journal about the significant effect exercise has on the muscles of the heart. The article pointed out that the heart is the most important organ in the body and that we have significant control over its effectiveness. The article further stressed the significance of developing a strong heart muscle. Its strength could be determined by counting how many times it beat while at rest. The stronger the muscle, the slower the resting heart rate. The stronger the muscle, the less often it has to contract to force the needed amount of blood to flow throughout the body. The article stated that the magic number for a heart to be at peak performance is a resting heart rate of forty beats a minute.

The article had so much more information than what my anatomy professor had. But they were both right. The heart makes it all happen.

The more I read additional medical literature, the more I committed to developing the strongest heart possible. I had planned to do lots of things before I grew too old to do them, and I wanted to find out what I could do to remain as active as possible for as long as possible. The more I read, the more I realized I wanted to die young, but at an old age. (In fact, I would like to peak at ninety.) The key to that "strongest heart as possible" was a lifestyle of exercise.

Eating Right

The more I read, the more I realized that even with my two new lifestyle changes of exercise and ideal weight, I was still missing one more essential strategy for fighting the aging progression. I hadn't examined the food I was eating. I was keeping my weight where I wanted it, but I was eating certain foods that would definitely cause blockage of my arteries. Unless I made a change, this would happen no matter what I weighed or how much I exercised.

I read about the significantly harmful effects of saturated fat and dietary cholesterol and began realizing that I needed to add one more strategy to my lifestyle if I wanted to stay as young physiologically as possible. I needed to cut out the foods that were causing plaque buildup in my arteries.

I read an article that pulled it all together for me. The statistics in that report were a real eye-opener, even for a vascular surgeon who had operated on the very problem I was reading about.

The article pointed out that more than half of Americans die as a result of problems of the arteries in their heart or brain. That figure stunned me. That's more than die from cancer. Then the report pointed out that almost all of these deaths are preventable. I wanted to know the details. I began to pull up more and more articles that explained that damage to your arteries caused by certain foods is the most common factor that causes you to age.

That is the moment I got serious about developing a complete, three-strategy lifestyle to keep me as young as possible, because I realized there were men in their seventies who looked and acted as if they were fifty-five and men who were fifty-five who looked and acted as if they were seventy.

That day, I committed to find out which foods I needed to avoid and which ones to eat.

Further reading showed that a particular cholesterol compound called Low Density Lipoprotein Cholesterol, or LDL, was the particle that gets into the walls of your arteries and sets up an inflammatory battleground, which either causes a clot in the artery or heals as a partial blockage of the artery.

I didn't want to believe it, but I discovered that Americans eat more saturated fat in cheese than in any other food. And the number one food that raises our LDL cholesterol is cheese. At that moment I decided to quit eating the food that Americans eat more of than anything else. Why? Because cheese causes the highest amount of what injures your arteries.

I will never forget that Christmas. All my patients knew that cheese was my favorite food. Every year, they brought me all kinds of cheeses, cheese balls, and cheese sticks. That Christmas, I didn't eat a bite of cheese. I love pizza, but I found I could order a cheese-less pizza. I admit, I do get some strange looks from the order taker, but I still enjoy a thin crust with small pieces of spiced grilled chicken and mushrooms and pineapple, with tomato sauce.

I wanted to read what the established medical journals said about a lifestyle of eating that avoids damage to arteries. I didn't want to rely on what I saw on television or what new fad diet or product some company or celebrity was selling. I wanted to read things that were proven by the double-blind studies the medical profession requires to acknowledge a finding as being factual. I wanted proof, not hype.

I read about red meat and dairy products like ice cream containing a large amount of saturated fat. You guessed it. I ate no more red meat, unless I was at a banquet where only steak was served. Then I would eat maybe half of it. I didn't want to become a fanatic, but I wanted my eating choices to be based on medical fact. Ice cream was probably the most difficult to give up, but fat-free yogurt made it a little easier.

Putting It All Together

Then a triple bonus: I read that not only the particular foods but also the combination of exercise and ideal weight worked together to keep my LDL Cholesterol down and protect my arteries. I'd uncovered the three lifestyle choices that would keep my body as young as possible. It did not matter what my birth certificate said; that indicated only my chronological age. I realized that after the age of forty, it isn't your chronological age that is important but your physiological age. And after all my reading, I realized that physiological age is determined by personal choice. I chose to commit to live as young of a physiological age as possible for the rest of my life.

I knew I was doing all the right things from a medical standpoint, but I didn't actually know medically if the changes I had made were paying off. It was only when I went to the Cooper Clinic in Dallas with one of my best friends that I found out.

My friend was in good shape. He exercised, but only somewhat, and his favorite food was barbecue pork. We both went through the clinic's complete physical examination program with blood work, treadmill and EKG testing, a colon examination, X-rays—the whole works.

When they hooked me up to cardiac monitors in preparation for a treadmill test, they had me lie down and then they left the room. Ten minutes later, they came back and said, "Are you alive?" My resting heart rate was 38. That was the first official medical indication that my cardiac training had paid off, but the real impact came at the end of the day when they discussed all they had found concerning my workup.

I will never forget how my doctor told me my cardiac status. Smiling, he said I was in the "above" 99th percentile group. He stressed it again by repeating, "Not *in* the 99th but *above* the 99th percentile." My cardiac status was better than over 99 percent of all people they had examined over the years in my age group. Then he told me something that made me realize all my work had paid off. "I just want you to know that, physiologically, you are a year younger than your friend. And he is eleven years younger than you—chronologically." That was when I realized that the Prescription for Life plan works, that it is medically based, and that I had passed the test.

Even though I'm a doctor, until I started my own quest to be as healthy as I could be, I'd never thought of aging "physiologically" or "chronologically." It was only at that moment that I realized that as you get older, you might as well throw away thinking about your chronological age. Your physiological age is what really counts. Your physiological age determines how well you live. I know pride is not something you should show, but I remember telling my friend, "I am a year younger, physiologically, than you, even though you are eleven years younger, chronologically, than me." I know I shouldn't, but I still remind him of that medical fact.

I began this journey when I was forty-two. I should have started sooner. I recently decided to share what I have learned about living younger longer. That is when I elected to do a current review of the medical literature and write it out in lay terms. That is what the Prescription for Life plan is all about. It's not about living longer, although you will add chronological years to your life span. It's not about death rate. It's much more important than adding x number of years to your life. *It's about the quality of your life.* I want quality. I want you to have that same quality. I want those over seventy to know the secret, the same as I want to share it with all the baby boomers. I want to tell young people in their twenties and thirties to realize that the sooner you begin the journey, the smoother the sailing. I want to share how to prevent damage to the arteries that ages you. I have come to the realization that I can save more lives with the Prescription for Life plan than I ever did in my entire surgical career. I shared with you several moments in my life when I made significant decisions that resulted in a younger age physiologically. I ask you to take just a *moment* right now and decide to fold those pants, place them back on the rack, and get started living younger.

Part 1

What You Need to Understand about the Aging Process

What you are about to learn is much more than a diet plan or how to lose weight or start an exercise program. It is more than getting your body to an ideal weight and maintaining that weight, and it's not just about preventing a heart attack or a stroke. It's not even just about the aging of your arteries.

The Prescription for Life plan also teaches you how to help prevent the major cancers. And you may not be diabetic or have high blood pressure now, but by the end of this book you will know how to prevent such conditions from occurring in your body.

In a nutshell, the goal is to live young physiologically—until you die at an old age chronologically. And the first step is to understand the aging process.

1

Your Course Determines Your Destination

It was mid-morning on Grand Cayman Island as I sat reading in a lounge chair in the shade of a casuarina pine. The sun was out, there was a slight breeze, and very few people were on the beach.

I looked up and saw him running like I had so many times before. I had watched him for several years, running the same route at least three days a week. He never wore a shirt, and the skin under his hairy shoulders was almost black from years of sun exposure. He was trim, muscular, and his stride was not all that fast, but it was consistent. I guessed him to be in his early sixties.

I got up out of my chair to trot along beside him and ask about his exercise routine. But when he saw me approaching, he stopped to talk. I couldn't believe how healthy and muscular he looked up close. He was Italian and had grown up in Italy, but he had worked in Saudi Arabia and Alaska for a worldwide contracting firm. He had been transferred to this island thirty years ago to help construct hotels and for the past ten years had stayed here in retirement. He was the epitome of good health.

I complimented him on his health, and that is all it took to turn on his "brag button." He immediately began telling me about his lifestyle. He ate mostly vegetables. He had weights and a stationary bicycle in his home. Three days a week, he was on his bike two hours in the morning. Three days a week, he jogged six miles on the beach. When he worked hotel construction on the beach, he would use his lunch break to swim a half mile straight out into the ocean. "Of course," he said with his Italian accent, "I had to swim the same distance back."

He had recently been tested physiologically. "I tell you my results," he said with his accent that made me smile. "I am seventy-five, but the machine say I am sixty-one. *I'm younger than I am.*" He flexed his arms and pulled his shoulders back. "Most of my friends my age on this island are old. They sit around and drink, and play cards, and watch television. Plus, they're fat—most of them."

Then he made the statement that made me admire him the most. "I want to be active when I die." He smiled and trotted off down the beach, waving with one hand without even glancing back.

That said it all. He didn't want to be active until a year before he died. He didn't want to be active until he died. He wanted to be active *when* he died. I don't know what the rest of his life is like, but I want to be like him physiologically.

With the Prescription for Life plan, you should be able to add seven to twelve years to your life expectancy, depending on your present condition. But what good is it to live longer if your mind doesn't recognize your friends or family? What good is it to extend your life if you are barely able to get around? What good is it to live more years if you are going to sit in a wheelchair and stare or be bedridden for the last part of your life?

No good at all—unless you are physiologically healthy during those extra years. And that's what this plan is all about. You can actually become younger physiologically than you are right now. With the Prescription for Life plan, when your chronological age is sixty-eight, your physiological age can be fifty.

You are about to begin a life-changing journey that will be worth far more than all the money you will ever have in your bank account. I like to use Charles Dickens's 1843 story, *A Christmas Carol*, as an illustration. As you probably recall, Ebenezer Scrooge is the principal character. Three ghosts come to him on Christmas Eve, and the last of the three is the ghost of Christmas "yet to come." This ghost takes Scrooge to a grave, where no one mourns the man who has died, where all he had in material goods is now for naught. The ghost reveals to Scrooge that this is his own future if his present course doesn't change. As you know, Scrooge makes a decision to change because he realizes in that *moment* what his future will be. He changes his course and turns his life around for the good.

This book will show you where you will end up if you continue on a wrong course. More than half of Americans are on that path, eating the wrong foods, enjoying life as couch potatoes, and not maintaining their ideal weight. They will hasten their demise if they stay on that course, if they choose not to change their direction.

It is sad to live in a world that dark—especially if you don't even know you need to change. You don't want to look back five years or ten years from now and say, "What might have been . . . if only."

Scrooge woke up the next morning realizing he could change. People do change. And no matter how good your lifestyle of eating, exercising, and weight control may be presently, even if it is great, it can get better.

If you're ready to make a change for the better, it will be helpful to find an accountability partner or group. Studies show that such support increases your exercise time by 20 percent. It works similarly in losing weight. Get a partner and you can both watch your physiological age decrease. Get a partner or join a group and commit to developing the three most important lifestyle strategies you can ever follow to remain as young as you possibly can.

Your journey begins here to get you on the right course, "yet to come."

2

Your Arteries Are the Cornerstone of the Aging Process

The aging process depends primarily on the condition of your arteries. If you remember nothing else I have said thus far, remember this: your arteries play a monumental role in the physiological aging of your body. The flow of blood through your body carries nutrients, oxygen, electrolytes, and other essentials that keep the body running like a new engine. That blood is pumped through your system by the heart and is carried by sixty thousand miles of arteries, plus veins.

The condition of the arteries determines how well the body is supplied with all it needs to function at 100 percent. As those arteries become damaged by certain cholesterol particles, the walls begin to respond by developing a battlefield to fight those foreign bodies, and either plaque buildup or inflammation results in a clot. Both events can cause the blood flow to either completely stop or become markedly decreased. The downstream area becomes starved for oxygen.

If the heart is involved, a portion of the muscle quits working and the remaining fibers are called on to carry an extra load of pumping your blood. The result is a less effective pump.

If the affected organ is the brain, that portion of brain tissue supplied by that particular artery quits working. If it is sudden, you have a stroke in which the part of the body supplied by that portion of the brain quits working immediately. If it is a slow blockage process, you could end up with what is called dementia, and slowly, over the years, you begin to forget, function slower, lose your reasoning, and finally lose your memory.

How Blockages Begin

The blockage process in an artery begins with certain cholesterol particles floating in the bloodstream. At different locations, usually where the artery divides or branches, there is turbulence in the blood flow. In such areas, these particles are pounded into the wall of the artery. They are forced through the inner lining and end up implanted within the wall. As time goes by, many more of these minute particles continue building up, and your body sends in special cells and a flood of fluid to begin fighting off these foreign bodies, which, of course, are not supposed to be there.

The result of such a battle is a partial or complete blockage. If it goes on long enough, even calcium can be deposited into the plaque formation. This is a silent process. It doesn't cause you any pain. It doesn't give you a headache or make your chest hurt. *It works quietly while you order extra cheese on your hamburger.*

Most people don't understand this process. You are getting ready to know exactly what is going on. I believe if you were standing in the middle of the railroad tracks and a freight train was coming, you would jump out of its way before it ran you over. I'm sounding the alarm so you can avoid that train with your health. When we finish, you won't be able to plead ignorance. You can do specific things every day for the rest of your life that will keep those blocking particles out of your bloodstream and those arteries youthful.

Let's look at the layers of an artery and see what happens when you eat the wrong foods. The thin inner layer is called the *intima*. Think of it as the protective portion of the arterial wall. It should be capable of keeping anything from getting through the inner lining and into the wall of the artery. Picture it as being made up of individual pieces of a thousand-piece jigsaw puzzle, each piece with a Teflon coating. This makes it smooth and slick, and nothing sticks to it or penetrates it. If you could magnify the intima, you would see that each of these interlocking cells is held together by little proteins, locked arm in arm. Think of these proteins as a line of soldiers that will not let anything penetrate through this lining.

Now let's go through that very thin inner lining and look at the next layer. This thicker, spongy layer is called the *media*. This is where the fighting takes place. Think of the media as the battleground of the aging process. This is where all kinds of things happen that determine whether you stay young or get older ahead of your chronological time frame. Even though so much fighting takes place in the media, the big problem is that we don't feel anything while the battle is going on.

If you were to hit your finger with a hammer, you would make all kinds of fuss. You would make sure that would never happen again. You would see the place the hammer hit immediately begin to swell. You most likely would put ice on it and elevate it to help prevent more swelling. But the problem with the damage that goes on in your arteries is that you are completely unaware it's happening, and you let it happen again and again.

Finally, we come to the *outer layer*, which is a thin, smooth covering that is fairly firm but pliable and doesn't really play a part in any of these problems.

You Are Only as Young as Your Arteries

Think about it a minute. If your arteries begin to age, you age. If you protect your arteries, you will, physiologically speaking, stop the clock. You can even turn your physiological age back quite a few years with some basic lifestyle changes that you can maintain the rest of your life.

Heart attacks, strokes, dementia, and erectile dysfunction are all caused by not protecting your arteries with a proper lifestyle. The same blockage happening in your heart is happening in the arteries to your kidneys, to your intestines, to the muscles in your legs, to every part of your body.

You may have absolutely no symptoms of blockage in your arteries, but I assure you that you have cholesterol deposits building up in your arteries. By the time patients present with EKG changes, or chest pain, or numbness going down their arm, it has already happened. We see the same thing with brains, when patients present with weakness, or numbness around their mouths, or dizziness.

It's an ongoing process because of your eating habits.

Many of these arteries are already 95 percent blocked. I have operated on many carotid arteries, the two main arteries going to the brain. Some have been 90 to 95 percent blocked without the patient ever having any symptoms. Their doctor just happened to find the blockage in a routine physical examination.

Don't wait for symptoms caused from the blockage of your arteries before you do something to prevent a stroke or heart attack. And for you men, the same goes for erectile dysfunction. Don't wait until it happens to decide you are going to protect your arteries.

Don't Let Your First Symptom Be Death

A few summers ago, I was at a fishing lodge in Alaska. A well-known individual lived nearby, and I had the opportunity to visit his home one afternoon. He appeared to be in excellent health except for being overweight. He said his blood pressure had always been normal. He had an almost constant, natural smile. Everything seemed great.

As I was standing by the lake before leaving, he mentioned he had experienced some occasional dizziness and that his doctor had started him on a blood thinner. I placed my right index and middle fingers on the left side of his neck to feel for his carotid pulse. The two carotid arteries, one on each side of the windpipe, are the major arteries feeding our brains. I wanted to see if I could feel turbulence in the blood flow. If dizziness happens to be the result of a partial blockage of the carotid artery, I can actually feel a vibration (physicians call that vibration a "thrill") as the blood squeezes through the partially blocked area. If there is partial blockage, that plaque can be removed to get normal flow going to the brain before a stroke occurs. If I felt such a vibration, I was going to tell him to go into town and have his arteries checked out.

I was surprised—not only did I not feel a "thrill" in his left carotid artery, but I didn't feel any pulse at all.

43

That was not good, because you can't operate on the artery after it is completely blocked. There is nothing surgically you can do to restore the blood flow to that side of the brain. My assumption was that he was supplying his entire brain from the remaining carotid. As he kept talking, I felt for the pulse in his right carotid. Nothing.

He had no blood flow through either of the major arteries to his brain. The brain has only four arteries supplying it, the two main carotids and two very small arteries in the back of the brain. I knew the only blood he was getting to his entire brain was from those two minute vertebral arteries. They normally carry less than 10 percent of total blood flow to the brain, but for him, they were carrying 100 percent.

I felt sick. The vehicles for the main blood supply to his brain were demolished. He had no symptoms except a little dizziness from time to time. Even though I realized nothing of significance could be done, I recommended he see his doctor again, concerning the dizziness. As I got into the boat to leave, I knew he had only a short time left on this earth.

He did see his doctor, but nothing could be suggested for him to do. Three months later, a friend informed me the gentleman had had a massive stroke and died.

The damage to his arteries had taken years and years to completely block the flow of life-giving blood to his brain. I tell you this story to emphasize you can have partial blockage of an artery in your body for years without any symptoms at all. His first symptom of dizziness was a warning that came too late for him to halt the process. Don't wait for symptoms. Even then, it may be too late.

And sometimes the first symptom is death.

You might think that gentleman in Alaska led a good life right up to the end, that he went quickly and didn't suffer so how he died might not be all that bad. But because of his lifestyle, his life ended way before it should have. He missed years and years that he could have spent with his family and friends—"if only."

Your Initial Symptom Could Be More Devastating Than Death

A stroke occurs when the blood supply to a particular part of the brain is suddenly halted. This can occur either by rupture of the artery, resulting in bleeding into the brain tissue, or by the artery becoming blocked, cutting off the oxygen to that area of the brain. Almost 90 percent of strokes are of the latter type, where arterial blockage is taking place due to plaque buildup. The stroke can be small and transient, called a transient ischemic attack (TIA), with temporary changes that disappear, or it can permanently change your mind and body. *Strokes are the leading cause of long-term disability in adults* and the fourth leading cause of death.

The moment you survive even a TIA you have *five times more chance of dying prematurely than someone who has not had a stroke.* Plus, within the next five years, *15 to 30 percent will have some form of permanent disability* due to a second stroke. Most strokes leave you with years of aftereffects. You may have slurred speech, be paralyzed on one entire side of your body, become bedridden, or develop dementia. You can live for years that way, affecting not only yourself but also loved ones who have to care for you.

Two million brain cells die each minute during a stroke. Six months after such a stroke, 20 percent of survivors who are sixty-five or older have difficulty speaking, while a third can't walk without assistance, and 25 percent end up in a nursing home.

I am trying to get your attention with all these statistics, but let me point out the most significant statistic concerning the blockage of arteries to your brain. *Sixty-one percent of stroke patients die or are back in the hospital within twelve months.* The American Heart Association informs us that stroke is the second leading cause of hospitalizations among the elderly. We are talking primarily about those over the age of sixty-five, but at any age when a stroke happens, only one phrase comes to my mind: "It's too late now." And one phrase you should never have to say to yourself is, "If only I had known." You are going to know—so that you can sow differently.

Too many people do not even realize they're at risk for a stroke. Last week I heard from a doctor who is practicing medicine in Africa for a six-month period. He is a typical American doctor, doing a very good service for humanity by helping out overseas. His numbers look pretty good except for low HDL Cholesterol. But he doesn't exercise, and he is about fifty pounds overweight. He said that one particular morning, as he was walking up the hill toward the hospital, he began having a little trouble with his balance. As he got near the hospital, rather than going to the usual ward to see his patients, he mysteriously found himself in the hospital laboratory. When he left the lab, he began having difficulty walking and was bumping against hedges, but he finally made it to the patient ward. He tried to tell the nurses something was wrong, but he had trouble coming up with the right words. His speech was slurred. It wasn't long before he was very dizzy and had double vision. All this happened within about thirty minutes. He was taken to a large city hospital where a CAT scan showed he had a small blockage in one of the arteries in his brain. Over the next forty-eight hours, his symptoms disappeared and he returned to normal. He went back to the hospital where he had been working, and within a few days he was carrying on as usual. Now his message to me was how thankful he was to be "back to normal," thankful that he had regained all his strength and was now able to do all the things he did before his "light stroke."

I hope I sounded the alarm by telling him not to be merely thankful that it was a light stroke and that he had fully recovered. I told him what he ought to be the *most* thankful for was that he'd received a warning signal.

The warning is this: someone who has had even a TIA is going to end up with a debilitating stroke sometime down the road if they don't do something about their lifestyle. Similar blockage is going on in the arteries of their heart, and if they don't do something about it right now, their fate and their future are already established.

Such individuals need to get to an ideal weight. They need to get an exercise program going, five to six days a week. Certain foods—as if they contain little sticks of dynamite—are imbedding trouble into the arteries to their brains, and they need to learn what is going on in their bodies and what they must eat and not eat to stop the impending danger. Anyone who has had any type of stroke is definitely a candidate for the Prescription for Life plan.

Aside from being rehospitalized for related causes, the sad reality is that within one year after having a stroke, 5 to 14 percent of patients end up having another stroke. And within five years following a stroke, 24 percent of women and 42 percent of men will have another stroke.

The American Stroke Association put together some stroke prevention plans and associated statistics that should get your attention. First, they recommend a similar diet to the one in the Prescription for Life plan—a diet low in saturated fat and in dairy products, such as cheese and whole milk, and high in fruits and vegetables. They also emphasize a normal body weight and exercise.

All this sounds familiar because stroke prevention is the same as heart attack prevention. Both events are caused by the same process in your arteries—resulting in either blockage or hemorrhage. Physiologically, a stroke is just a heart attack in the brain.

Stroke is the fourth most common cause of death among Americans. Of individuals who survive a stroke, 20 percent remain in a hospital or nursing home or recovery institution for three months. Think about how depressing that can get. But this is the statistic that scares me. This is the one I tell anyone I know who has had a stroke. I tell them as a "moment" of thought to encourage them to do something to get rid of the dynamite.

Fifteen to 30 percent of people who survive a stroke become permanently disabled.

You don't want to wait until you have a stroke to think about how lifestyle change is the major factor in preventing a stroke.

Science tells us that your actions rely on knowledge. You are much more likely to enact change in your lifestyle if you understand what happens in your body. I firmly believe that if you know what happens when you put bites of certain foods into your system, you will be much less likely to put that particular food into your mouth again. You won't need a medical degree to understand this, but by the time you are finished with this book, I assure you that you will equate the condition of your arteries with the process of aging.

The Arterial Path through Your Body

Because the physiological aging process is the result of damage to the walls of your arteries, I want to take you on a short anatomical trip covering your major arteries so you will understand the impact of how you decide to live.

Let's start with the heart. It is the most important of the organs because that is how physicians determine that someone is dead: the patient's heart stops beating. When a doctor looks at an EKG monitor, he or she can see each beat of an active heart. But when there is a straight line across the screen, there is no cardiac activity. At that moment, the patient is pronounced dead. It's not when the kidneys shut down, or when the intestines quit working, or when the liver backs up bile into the body. Death is determined when the heart quits beating. The amount of blood flowing through the arteries of that heart muscle is the most significant factor to the function of the heart.

The aorta is the main large artery coming out of the heart. The carotid arteries, feeding the brain, branch off just past the heart. The aorta then passes through the chest on down through the abdomen, dividing to enter each leg.

Whenever I hear someone talk about brain damage, I think of that gentleman in Alaska, the one I was hoping had only a partial blockage of his carotid arteries in his neck so it could be surgically corrected. Your carotid is about the size of your index finger. I have operated on them following a stroke or after discovering a partial blockage. In surgery, with the artery open, I have found all degrees of the aging process going on. When I cut it open to clean it out, there may be a soft plaque that feels like butter blocking 80 percent of the artery. It may have no calcium in it at all. Another patient may have a 95 percent blockage, and the process of the obstruction may have been going on so long that calcium has been laid down throughout the plaque. After I take it out and hold it in my fingers, it feels like bone.

You don't have to be even half smart to realize that you want to do everything possible to prevent having anything like a piece of bone stuck inside the main source of blood supply to your brain.

As we look beyond the large carotid, we see thousands of smaller arteries within the brain. Visualize some of them beginning to block. Many times, the result is dementia. Think about the aging process going on in these smaller arteries the next time you forget where you left your car keys or can't remember someone's name.

Soon after the aorta enters the abdomen, the artery that feeds our small intestine comes directly off that main aorta. Just below it are the renal arteries, which supply the kidneys. The partial blockage of these is one of the causes of high blood pressure. Any organ that doesn't get sufficient blood supply doesn't function properly.

Moving lower in males, you come to the penile artery. The same process that causes blockage in the arteries of the heart causes blockage in the arteries supplying the penis. And just like that kidney, the penis does not function properly without good blood supply. Partial blockage of the penile artery is the most significant cause of erectile dysfunction. Recent studies in the medical literature show a correlation between erectile dysfunction and disease in the heart arteries. Some of these studies are showing that up to a fourth of the time, erectile dysfunction is a warning sign that there are blockages in the arteries of your heart.

Later in this book, there is an entire section on erectile dysfunction—preventing it, reversing it. But now I want to emphasize the possible connection between blocked arteries and this condition that is affecting so many men. It has to be a common problem if you can't turn on the television without seeing an advertisement about it.

A research article published in the medical journal *Circulation* talks about the relationship between erectile dysfunction and heart disease in patients who have a high risk for heart disease. The title of the paper is "Erectile Dysfunction Predicts Cardiovascular Events in High-Risk Patients." It addresses high-risk patients, but the lesson to be learned is this: if you do have erectile dysfunction, you need to be aware of the possibility that it is caused by a partial blockage of the penile artery. Blood flow tests can be performed to show significant blockage, but the main idea is to *prevent* it from ever happening by following the Prescription for Life plan. Such blockage can be a significant warning flag that the same blockage process may be going on in the arteries of your heart, which can be fatal.

This will be discussed in more detail later, but the main point you need to carry away from this discussion is the fact that if you have blockage of arteries in one area of your body, you most likely have it in multiple places throughout your body.

Let me give you an example of this "multiple artery problem." At the age of eighty-seven, my father developed a little chest pain. He had never had any symptoms prior to that day. After he was examined, he had an emergency operation to bypass the blockage that had been forming in that artery in his heart for years. It was a successful procedure, but four years later he began having abdominal pain. A surgeon performed another emergency operation in his abdomen and found that the artery supplying his small intestine was completely blocked and his small bowel had died. All the surgeon could do was sew my father's abdomen back together. That blockage of the main artery to his small intestine had been forming for years.

The partial blockage of the artery in his heart preceded the complete blockage of the artery to his intestines. The process was taking place throughout his body, not just with his heart. There were no symptoms warning him of what was happening.

Similar to how blockage of the artery to the kidney does not let the kidney function normally, and how blockage of the artery to the heart keeps the heart muscle from performing properly, and how blockage of the artery in the neck keeps the brain from functioning properly, the complete blockage of the artery leading to the small intestine caused my father's intestines to turn necrotic and quit functioning. Nothing could be done to save the intestine, and my father died post-op. If he had known there were things he could have been doing to prevent blockage of his arteries, he would have done them.

If *I* had known the Prescription for Life plan back then, he would not have lived in a way that blocked the artery to his small intestine. I would have made sure he knew what to eat. I would have had him begin something I never saw him do—exercise. He wasn't obese, but he was overweight. I would have encouraged him to get down to his ideal weight.

Yes, I wish I had known then what I know now.

The aging process that took my father is the aging process you are going to avoid by developing a new lifestyle to give you physical quality for the rest of your life.

The Drool Factor

Let's take a minute to *not* talk about death. Let's concentrate on one of the most important reasons for developing the Prescription for Life way of living. The problem usually begins several years before you die. It is a process of intellectual deterioration called *dementia*, and I want you to fully understand how to prevent what may be the worst problem of aging. I think it is worse than death, because suffering with dementia can last a long, terrible, devastating period of time.

Many underlying causes play a part in developing dementia, but a significant cause is a decrease in blood flow through arteries leading to and throughout the brain. Some people call its results the "drool factor." Others call it the "sunset club syndrome." To me, avoiding dementia is one of the major reasons to commit to the Prescription for Life plan. So many times, the aging process nears its end with a person's body alive but their mind "gone." I am sure you have elderly friends, or even parents, who have no idea who you are when you visit them. They can carry on a conversation about the past very exactly but have no idea about today. This is the prime example of what you want to avoid by developing a better lifestyle. Now is the *moment* of realization that you want quality years up to the end of your life, no matter when that may be.

Alzheimer's is a form of dementia and a growing problem in America. In fact, it is now the sixth leading cause of death. If you categorize it by age group, in people over sixty-five it is the fifth leading cause of death. It causes more deaths than diabetes.

I have had individuals tell me, "I don't really want to live to be ninety. I've seen too many people in nursing homes, sitting in chairs, staring. I don't want to be one of them."

No matter how old you live to be, you do not want those last years to end up with you not knowing what day it is, or where you are, or who in the world is talking to you. You don't want to have any form of dementia, whether Alzheimer's or arteriosclerotic dementia. You want to be like the seventy-five-year-old Italian jogger I met on the beach, who said, "I want to be active when I die." We should all want the same—to still be both physically and mentally active when we die.

Alzheimer's is a common disorder among the elderly. The good news is that it is found in only about 1 percent of individuals sixty to sixty-five years old. The bad news is that the percentage doubles every five years until Alzheimer's is found in more than 40 percent of individuals over the age of eighty-five. Those are terrible odds. Here is an even worse statistic: Alzheimer's currently is affecting over 5.6 million people in the United States and is expected to be triple that number before 2050.

When talking about maintaining the quality of your life, dementia is the huge brick wall. When people make plans for their later years, many will have to include stays in a nursing home or other means of care because their minds will not be functioning at their full potential.

However, dementia can be prevented. The Prescription for Life plan path is the one to take. There are two main subtypes of dementia: vascular dementia and Alzheimer's disease. The vascular risks we have been discussing also apply to vascular dementia and even partially to Alzheimer's disease. Look at it this way: when you block portions of the arteries in your brain, you are decreasing the blood flow through that vessel. If you're drinking a glass of water through a straw and you crimp that straw, the flow of water diminishes. When you consider all the nutrients necessary to keeping the brain's memory functioning properly, your brain tissue is going to falter if you block a significant portion of blood flow.

The bottom line is that arterial aging is a major cause of memory loss.

An article in the *Journal of Nutrition, Health and Aging* had lots of food for thought. It reviewed several studies, including the Rotterdam Study, in which almost eight thousand individuals fifty-five or older were followed. The overall results found an association between certain foods individuals ate and the incidence of dementia. It was found that total fat, saturated fat, and dietary cholesterol intake increased the risk of dementia, especially of vascular dementia. Another journal article pointed out similar findings, where there is a correlation between the amount of saturated fat consumed and the prevalence of Alzheimer's disease among individuals over the age of sixty-five.

A third journal article emphasizes the significance of your LDL Cholesterol level. In this book, you will be learning how eating the wrong foods results in an elevation of the LDL and that this elevation is related to developing Alzheimer's.

The study consisted of two groups of patients. One group had Alzheimer's and the other group did not. The patients with Alzheimer's disease had higher levels of LDL Cholesterol than patients who were in the non-Alzheimer's control group. That result was mainly due to the bad foods eaten by the Alzheimer's group versus the good foods eaten by the non-Alzheimer's group.

The Prescription for Life plan will result in your not only living longer but also living with a better quality of life, decreasing your worry about the "drool factor."

But first, let's learn more about cholesterol.

3

Understanding Cholesterol
Is Essential

Several years ago I bought a new four-wheel drive Audi, which gets me through the snow in the wintertime. Six months later, I was driving along the Blue Ridge Parkway when a red light came on. It said "check engine." I immediately pulled over and got the owner's manual out of the glove compartment. Page 47 stated that I should not drive the car for a prolonged period of time but should have it checked at the dealership as soon as possible.

I immediately took it in, and they drained the "new engine oil" and replaced it with the standard kind. I thought I had been doing everything I was supposed to do, but I had not realized at what mileage I was supposed to have the initial oil changed.

Your cholesterol numbers are like warning lights for your body. You need to learn what it means when they are on and flashing.

Cholesterol is a fatty substance that exists in the outer layer of every cell in your body, maintaining each cell's membrane. It is involved in the production of sex hormones, as well as hormones released by your adrenal glands. It insulates nerve fibers. It is significant in the metabolism of certain vitamins, including A, D, and E. It is essential to your body. Cholesterol is carried through the bloodstream combined with a protein. The structure of the cholesterol with the protein is a molecule called a lipoprotein. There are two main types of lipoproteins, both of which you will recognize on your lab report as Low Density Lipoprotein and High Density Lipoprotein, or LDL and HDL.

You may think you are doing everything possible to keep your engine running like the owner's manual instructs. You may be eating free-range meat and everything organic. You may take vitamins or all kinds of supplements. You may take an aspirin a day because you heard it can keep you from having a heart attack. You may be doing all you know to do, but you don't know from a medical standpoint that some of the things you routinely eat every day may be harming you a thousand times more than all of the "supplemental medicines" you are taking. As a medical fact, some of your favorite foods may be the ones causing the most damage.

The probability is that your check engine light—in the form of your cholesterol levels—is on and flashing, and like most Americans you haven't noticed, or if you have, you haven't done much about it. So many take great care of their car but not of their body.

Stepping aside from specifics about cholesterol for a moment, I want to say that this plan teaches you not to wait for the red light to go on. The Prescription for Life plan is not about treatment; it is about *prevention*.

Let me tell you a little secret—why you don't want to wait on symptoms before beginning to do something about protecting your arteries. I say it's a secret, because hardly anyone talks about it though it comes out of the medical literature. *Eighty-five percent of everyone over the age of fifty has some* significant *blockage in the arteries of their heart, without experiencing any symptoms.*

That is a scary statement. They haven't had the first pain in their chest. They haven't had any undue shortness of breath. They haven't experienced any pain shooting down their left arm. That report is saying that most individuals over fifty have significant blockages in their coronary arteries yet don't even know it because there are no *symptomatic* red lights warning them.

Two-thirds of the time, the first symptom of artery blockage is a heart attack. There are no bells or whistles before it happens. People are going along routinely, and then they have a heart attack.

And that first attack can be fatal. Now, that's bad enough, but what if you do wait until you have that first symptom, that first attack? What are your chances then? Even if you survive your first heart attack, you are six times more likely to have another one than someone who has never had such an attack.

Don't wait until you have symptoms from the blockage of your arteries. Begin working right now on preventing the cause of the aging of your arteries. And even if you have a first attack, a second attack is preventable and you can learn how to avoid it.

Aging of the arteries starts at a much younger age than most people think. By the age of twelve, 70 percent of children have microscopic fatty deposits in their arteries. Studies of twenty-five-year-old individuals who were killed in battle or died in traffic accidents show that up to 60 percent of them already had some visual evidence that this process was taking place in their arteries.

Abnormal cholesterol numbers are great warning lights, better than attacks. Get your physician to order your blood lipids and learn what each means. Get your owner's manual out and see how your numbers line up to keep your motor running for hundreds of thousands more miles.

Understanding Your Blood Lipid Report

When your physician gives you your lipid profile results, you will see your Total Cholesterol, LDL Cholesterol, HDL Cholesterol, HDL/Total Cholesterol ratio, and triglyceride results. Your doctor will probably tell you that your Total Cholesterol should be below 200, that your LDL Cholesterol should be below 100, and that your HDL Cholesterol should be above 40 if you are male and above 50 if you are female. Your HDL/Total Cholesterol ratio should be below 3.5, and your doctor will probably tell you your triglycerides should be below 150.

Triglyceride molecules start out combined with proteins and break away from them, resulting in your triglyceride number on that report. Triglycerides represent the fat in your body. They are either made in the body or eaten as fat in your food. Calories that are eaten but not used are converted into triglycerides and stored in fat cells. When your body needs energy and there is no food source, triglycerides are released from those fat cells and used for energy. We will not concentrate so much on the triglycerides, because if you do what the Prescription for Life plan says to do, your triglycerides will come down to normal as your cholesterol numbers are corrected.

Total Cholesterol

Both good (HDL) and bad (LDL) cholesterol particles are floating around in your blood. You get cholesterol primarily from two places: your liver produces it and you eat it in certain foods. The liver produces all the cholesterol you need for your body to function. The excess comes from the wrong foods you eat.

When people talk about their "cholesterol" number, they're usually referring to what's called Total Cholesterol. When you think of Total Cholesterol, think of adding the LDL and HDL together. You will realize the two don't quite add up to the total number, but that is because additional particles are not listed.

Let's see what the medical literature has to say about the significance of your Total Cholesterol number. A report in the *Journal of the American Medical Association* studied the life expectancy of younger men who had a favorable Total Cholesterol level compared to men of the same age who had a significantly unfavorable Total Cholesterol level. The study concluded that the men who had the favorable, lower level of Total Cholesterol had a life expectancy of 3.8 to 8.7 years longer than the ones with the unfavorable, higher level of Total Cholesterol. There was a continuous, proportional relationship between the amount of Total Cholesterol and the life expectancy difference.

Those figures alone give you a huge insight into the importance of controlling what you are doing to your body. High Total Cholesterol spells danger for you. Remember 3.8 to 8.7 years the next time you think about your cholesterol report.

The next step in understanding your numbers is to realize that the Total Cholesterol is the sum of a whole lot of "bad" cholesterol as well as a small amount of "good" cholesterol. When your Total Cholesterol number is high, the biggest number is the "bad" kind of cholesterol. There are not as many of the "good" HDL particles, but they are much more powerful than the "bad" LDL particles. A little increase of the "good" is as important as a larger decrease of the "bad."

Understanding the significance of your Total Cholesterol, LDL Cholesterol, and HDL Cholesterol numbers enables you to understand what each cholesterol particle is doing to your body physiologically. Then you'll want to begin learning which foods cause the aging process and which ones protect against it. And once you understand what foods elevate your "lethal" LDL Cholesterol and what foods lower your "hero" HDL Cholesterol, getting the cholesterol numbers you need becomes almost too easy because you realize why you shouldn't be eating certain foods. It is almost like cheating.

The numbers you will shoot for with the Prescription for Life plan will be a Total Cholesterol of 200, LDL Cholesterol of 100, and an HDL/Total Cholesterol ratio of less than 3.5. However, you're not just shooting for a number; you're shooting for the kind of lifestyle that gets you to that number. Merely taking a pill is not the answer. It is not the same as getting your Total Cholesterol to 200 by eating properly, developing an ideal weight, and exercising routinely. There are no shortcuts in beating the aging process. A pill should be a *supplement*, not a *treatment*.

LDL Cholesterol

LDL stands for Low Density Lipoprotein Cholesterol. Think of the *L* as standing for "lethal," because it is. LDL is the bad cholesterol. If LDL levels get too high, bad cholesterol gets into the walls of your arteries, and the aging process accelerates. The resulting danger is the inflammation and narrowing of arteries throughout your body.

Years of medical research show a causative link between high cholesterol and heart disease. The term "high cholesterol" actually refers to high LDL Cholesterol, because those are the cholesterol particles that make up most of your total cholesterol number. Back in 1985, the National Heart, Lung, and Blood Institute made the direct correlation between high blood cholesterol and heart attacks. They published the *National Cholesterol Education Program* to point out the danger of LDL Cholesterol and to show that reducing your LDL Cholesterol reduces your risk for blockage of your arteries, with a corresponding reduction of heart attacks. That was a good basis in 1985 for progressing to what we know today.

THE SPLINTER SYNDROME

Getting a splinter in your finger is the best illustration to show what happens when LDL Cholesterol gets into the walls of your arteries. I call the reactive process that takes place the *Splinter Syndrome*. The skin where the splinter is embedded begins to swell and turn red. The surrounding tissue considers that splinter a "foreign body," and if the splinter does not come out, your body's natural response is to develop a wall of scarring tissue around it.

The initial swelling around the splinter is the result of the body pouring fluid into the area. The fluid is filled with soldier-type cells, called macrophages, that attack the splinter. Many times there is even bleeding into this swollen battlefield. The finger turns red and more swollen. Finally, one of two things happens. The resulting inflammation can be so fierce that it swells and the fluid breaks through the skin and drains out. An example of this is a boil that ruptures and drains from the battleground tissue to the outside. Or, after the battle against the foreign body splinter reaches its height, healing begins to take place. The body sends cells called fibroblasts that begin to lay down fibers that join together to form a healing scar throughout the battlefield.

This scar tissue is not the normal kind of tissue that was once there. Scar tissue is firmer and harder and is not pliable. You

can palpate the thickened, hardened area of scar tissue forming just under the skin's surface. And that scar remains—fixed,
thickened, firm, hard, and swollen. And if another splinter enters
the skin at that same area, another battle takes place, and the
resulting scar area gets larger and larger. After repeated battles,
calcium can become a part of the healing, and the plaque buildup
is even firmer and harder.

LDL Cholesterol Is the Splinter

A similar process is happening in the walls of your arteries.
LDL Cholesterol is the splinter that gets through the lining of
the artery and into the *media*, the middle portion of the arterial
wall. However, there is a difference between getting a splinter
stuck in your finger and getting an LDL Cholesterol splinter
stuck in the wall of your artery.

If you stick your hand into the middle of a thornbush and
get stuck, you won't stick it in again because you felt the pain
of the prick. The problem with the LDL Cholesterol Splinter
Syndrome is that you don't feel the splinters going into your
arteries. These splinters get through the lining wall of your
arteries and cause the battle to begin. The battleground you
visualize within the tissue of your finger is very similar to the
battleground within the middle part of the wall of your artery.
And similar to the reaction to the splinter in your finger is the
reaction that begins within the wall of your artery. The area
can become so inflamed that there is bleeding with the inflammatory reaction, and it can rupture through the lining into the
lumen of the artery. A clot forms and plugs the entire artery
at that point.

Or the arterial wall can stay intact and the splinter battleground ends in a healing process. But the scars of battle remain. The enlarged scar formation protrudes into the lumen

of the artery, and the result is a partial blockage of the flow of blood through that area (like crimping a straw). This is what is commonly referred to as plaque buildup. The next time an LDL Cholesterol splinter gets stuck in the same area, the process repeats itself. The secondary battleground either pops open and causes a clot to form inside the artery, or it can heal again and bulge even more into the inside of the artery. The result is more plaque buildup. This secondary plaque protrudes even farther into the lumen of the artery, causing the flow of blood to be even less to the heart muscle downstream.

Your only real protection is to keep the LDL Cholesterol splinters from getting into your bloodstream, and the best defense is avoiding three types of food. The first and major cause of LDL Cholesterol elevation is *saturated fat*. The foods we eat in America are full of saturated fat. It is found in red meat and cheese and other dairy products, as well as in pies, pastries, cakes—and in many more foods as well. The second cause of raised LDL Cholesterol is called *trans fat*, which is found mainly in pastries and cakes and wrapped foods that need a long shelf life. Trans fat is so bad that the government has recently outlawed it. The third is *dietary cholesterol*, which you find in foods such as egg yolks and butter.

It is imperative to keep your LDL Cholesterol low. But how you get there is more important than just getting the numbers down. You can be fooled if you're only looking at the numbers. Taking medication alone, without lifestyle changes, isn't a guarantee that you are doing all you can to protect your arteries. You should work on your LDL score as you would your golf score—the lower the better.

With the Prescription for Life plan, you learn which foods you commonly eat that contain saturated fat, trans fat, and dietary cholesterol. You are going to implant a picture of these "foods to avoid" deep within your mind. As a matter of fact, you will be able to recite them from memory before long.

HDL Cholesterol

The other side of the coin from the lethal LDL Cholesterol is the HDL Cholesterol. It is called the High Density Lipoprotein Cholesterol. Think of the *H* as standing for "hero" or "healthy." This is the good cholesterol you will be attempting to get as high as possible. It actually fights the lethal LDL Cholesterol. The tricky part is that, proportionally, you always have a lot more LDL Cholesterol particles than HDL Cholesterol particles. Think of football or baseball scores when thinking HDL. The higher the better.

It doesn't seem quite fair to men, but women tend to have more HDL than men. If a man's HDL is below 40 and a woman's is below 50, it's a definite red flag that must be addressed. Having such low HDL numbers is medically similar to being obese, to smoking, or to having diabetes or high blood pressure.

Exercise and weight loss are the two most important factors that affect your HDL Cholesterol. While you concentrate on the idea that certain foods raise your LDL Cholesterol, begin thinking of exercising and weight loss for getting your HDL higher.

HDL Cholesterol protects you by battling the LDL Cholesterol. Here is an easy way to visualize how it works. Think of an HDL Cholesterol particle as a police car that floats through the bloodstream, looking for LDL Cholesterol criminals. Imagine the HDL Cholesterol police car pulling up to an area where LDL Cholesterol "splinters" are getting into the wall of an artery. The HDL police car picks up several splinters and carries them to the liver and deposits them there to be disposed of. The liver takes the LDL Cholesterol particles and passes them out of the body in the bile. While the liver is working to place this excess LDL Cholesterol into the process of forming bile, the High Density Lipoprotein "police car" particle is on its way back to the arteries, where it picks up some more LDL Cholesterol to transport back to the liver.

You want as many HDL Cholesterol "police cars" as you can have. You will learn later how exercise and weight loss get as many HDL Cholesterol particles into your bloodstream as possible.

HDL/Total Cholesterol Ratio

Imagine a gang of hoodlums rioting, turning over cars, breaking store windows, stealing, fighting, and harming innocent citizens. How many police officers would you want to send in to pick up as many of the hoodlums as possible? Obviously, the more police officers you have per hoodlum the better. At the very least, you would want a certain minimum ratio of police officers per hoodlum to be safe.

That same logic applies to your HDL/Total Cholesterol ratio. Even more important than knowing your Total Cholesterol number or your single LDL Cholesterol number is looking at how much "hero" HDL Cholesterol you have in comparison to your Total Cholesterol. The higher your number of HDL particles within your Total Cholesterol number, the more police cars in proportion to fewer splinters.

This ratio is significant because it combines the interworking of both LDL and HDL Cholesterol. The lower your LDL and the higher your HDL, the better that ratio number will be. You figure your HDL/Total Cholesterol ratio by dividing your Total

Cholesterol number by your HDL Cholesterol number. The Prescription for Life plan uses 3.5 as the cut-off number. You want your ratio to be *below* 3.5. The importance of a low ratio number is backed up by multiple studies in medical literature. They show that eating foods high in saturated fat, trans fat, and dietary cholesterol has a negative effect on that ratio, while exercise and weight loss have a positive effect.

The significance of knowing your HDL/Total Cholesterol ratio is that you have two avenues to improve it.

1. *Lower* your lethal LDL Cholesterol—and that is primarily by avoiding foods with the bad fats.
2. *Raise* your hero HDL Cholesterol—and that is by losing weight and exercising.

The Three Good Fats

The bad fats are saturated fat, trans fat, and dietary cholesterol. Three good fats improve your HDL/Total Cholesterol ratio. These are monounsaturated fat, polyunsaturated fat, and omega-3 fat.

The best examples of foods that contain these good fats are olives, nuts, and fish. Even though such foods contain some saturated fat, the "good threes" outweigh the danger and actually protect your arteries.

You will notice this if you look at the Nutrition Facts box on a regular peanut butter jar. You will see 2.5 grams of saturated fat. That is way over the zero target and 0.5 absolute limit you will learn about later. However, you will see Total Fat at 16 grams, and the vast majority of that is from the "good threes" fat category. These help raise your HDL and overall protection.

Case Studies in Cholesterol

John

He was friendly as can be, and everybody liked to be around him. He had no history of heart disease in his family, and he was on no medication. But John was forty pounds overweight with a high Total Cholesterol count, and he was a true couch potato.

It was a blustery January evening, one so cold you wouldn't want to take a single step outside if you didn't have to. On the coffee table by the sofa where he was lounging were several empty wrappers from cheese crackers, two chocolate candy bars, and half a bowl of multicolored candies, which he was eating only two at a time.

John felt a little pain in his chest and mentioned it to his wife. She didn't think much about it, and they both kept watching television. About thirty minutes later, it hit him again. He abruptly got up from the sofa and quite sternly informed her he was going to the ER. She ran to get her coat out of the bedroom closet, but by the time she got back to the front hall he was driving out the driveway through the snow without her. The pain had suddenly become so severe that he was afraid he was going to die on the spot. He didn't even take time to get his coat. All he could think of was getting to the hospital before he passed out.

As John was briskly walking up to the admitting clerk at the ER, he suddenly fell, unconscious. They immediately put him on a stretcher, shocked his heart, and pumped medication into his veins. Within hours, a stent was placed in his blocked left coronary artery. If he had left home two minutes later, he would have died in his car on the way to the hospital. But John was a survivor.

At least for the time being.

His doctor informed him his cholesterol was elevated and handed him a booklet about what his diet should be. She told him to lose some weight and that it would be good if he started exercising. John listened to the advice, but all he could think about was his pilot's license. He flew a small bush plane for Alaskan hunters for his livelihood, and his biggest concern was how to keep his business going. The question in his mind was whether he was going to lose his license because of his heart attack.

It never occurred to John that the disease that caused his near-death event was a continuing process. It never occurred to him that the food he had been putting into his stomach was the cause of his heart attack. He didn't realize that even though he had one heart artery blocked off, he had multiple additional heart arteries that could also be blocked purely because of his lifestyle of poor eating, no exercising, and being overweight.

Most of all, he didn't realize that, beginning right then, he could do something to prevent another heart attack—one that could prove fatal.

John's doctor never stressed the three factors that could stop the deadly process going on in his body—getting thin, getting his LDL Cholesterol below 100, and exercising.

He was given a pamphlet.

Informed—so to speak.

The rest was up to him.

No one told John what a report of the American College of Cardiology/American Heart Association Task Force of Practice Guidelines stated. If he read one of the key statements in the article, he would change his thinking—because it spoke specifically about first heart attacks like his. It said that after having a first heart attack at age forty or older, 23 percent of women and 18 percent of men die within one year and that those death rates jump up—43 percent of women and 33 percent of men will expire within five years because of that initial heart attack.

John just didn't know. It wasn't real to him that what blocked one artery would continue to block others in his body unless he did something to halt the process in its tracks.

I saw John several months after his event. "What do you think I ought to be doing?" he asked me, "because I sure don't want to go through that again. You know how a lot of people who have gone through a near-death experience tell how they saw a light? You know, a light of heaven? Well, I didn't see a light." He said it scared him nearly to death going into that emergency room and blacking out. I spent over an hour informing him what he should be doing to prevent further disease to the other arteries in his heart.

As I talked to him, he was attentive, asked a lot of questions, made some notes, and thanked me for my concern about him, not only as a doctor but also as a friend. But within an hour, he was eating some of the exact foods I had just explained would plug his heart arteries again. Will he make it after a second attack? I don't know, but it doesn't seem to concern him all that much. At least, it doesn't concern him enough to change his lifestyle right now.

Eric

Eric was thirty-eight years old and a college football coach. He had been a star quarterback himself and was as dedicated a young man as you can find. He had an extremely nice wife and two little children. His team had recently won a national championship, which was great to have accomplished, but that made a workaholic out of all the coaches in preparation for next season.

Eric's father had died of a heart attack at age fifty-eight, but no one else in his family had any history of heart disease. Eric was trim, in shape, and ran five miles almost every day. Even during football season, he and three of the other coaches used their lunchtime for a run. If you looked at him and knew how active he was, you thought he was in the best physical condition possible.

Eric's blood pressure was normal, he ate the usual foods, and he had zero concern, health-wise. Zero concern, that is, until he happened to get a blood test at the college infirmary. And the only reason he did that was because one of the coaches he ran with decided all four of them should stop there to get blood work done free of charge.

That was when Eric came to me with his results: Total Cholesterol—262, LDL Cholesterol—178, and HDL Cholesterol—71.

The school doctor informed him it was essential to get his cholesterol down, and if he could not do it with a change in lifestyle, he would have to start on medication. His doctor explained that because of his family history, he was a prime candidate for a heart attack.

Eric was obviously shaken. He was thinking mostly about his young daughters, his wife, and his dad dying so young. He couldn't believe it. He was in great shape, a jogger, and not an ounce overweight. He had never thought about having a health problem.

John and Eric are typical of so many Americans. But let's look at how each of them handled his situation, and you will see the secret to changing your own life for the better. It's a great secret to learn.

"I will do anything to keep from having a heart attack like my father had," Eric, the football coach, said. "I want to be around for my wife and children." He looked at me as earnestly as I have ever seen any patient look. "I will set any goal, do whatever it takes to keep from dying early in life."

Eric saw his problem and committed to do something about it. I explained that he definitely had to get his LDL Cholesterol down. That would lower his Total Cholesterol also. With the history of his father dying from a heart attack and his cholesterol so extremely elevated, he needed to look at his situation as urgent. He would have to go extreme on his new eating strategy or begin medication now.

He decided to begin the Prescription for Life plan for an eight-week trial and then decide about his medication. We went over what foods he should eat and which ones to avoid. We added some specifics to his exercise with plans to get his heart rate elevated and sustained for thirty minutes at a time, and we planned to wait two months to repeat his lipid studies.

Eric became near fanatical about his eating habits. The other coaches told me they couldn't get him to eat a single French fry, and fries had been one of his favorite foods. He wouldn't get near cheese and avoided red meat like it was a poison. He ate a lot of fruit, loads of vegetables, and salads.

At the end of two months, the school doctor called me with Eric's lipid profile. His LDL was 98 and all of his cholesterol numbers and ratio were completely normal.

I believed Eric when he said he was committed to his new lifestyle—for the rest of his life. He never had to start on the medication, which, again, he would have had to take for the rest of his life. He will never have to be concerned with the possible side effects of that medicine as the years pass. He is in control. With such a good report in hand, I called the football field house and asked to speak with Eric. He couldn't come to the phone right then; he was exercising.

One year later, John is still forty pounds overweight, with a high Total Cholesterol count. His LDL is high and his HDL is low. He remains as friendly as can be. Everybody likes to be around him. He still keeps a bowl of candy on the table beside his sofa. He still eats only two pieces at a time. I wish he realized he could be around a lot longer—if he weren't still a true couch potato.

I kept asking myself why there are Erics and why there are Johns. And was there anything more I could do to instruct people like Eric and help people like John. Looking back on my surgical career, I saw the countless individual lives I had the privilege to make better, prolong, or save. And it is comforting to realize the number of people I helped. But I also realized I could help a hundred- or thousandfold more by simply figuring out a plan that would reach both the Erics and the Johns. I came to understand that a big part of why my friends and patients did not take proper care of their bodies is simply because they did not fully comprehend what was going on inside their bodies. They didn't have the knowledge to see what their future health was going to be.

People have a difficult time correlating what they are eating with how that one specific bite of food is affecting the arteries in different parts of their bodies. They don't grasp the significance of being twenty pounds overweight or two hundred pounds overweight. They don't know the importance of exercise in their overall lifestyle. They seem to accept their aging process but do not understand that they have a huge opportunity to control that aging.

John and Eric each put a different "face" on the need. They both need to know the proper plan. And, again, that is why the Prescription for Life plan was conceived. I want to save lives. I want to be able to help you remain healthy and live younger than you are today.

Warning Signs

Do you recall the numbers given by the American Heart Association? Within five years after having their first heart attack, 43 percent of women and 33 percent of men will expire. That is unless they do something about their lifestyle. These are people who, for years, had no idea there was a significant blockage problem going on in their arteries. They never acknowledged they needed to change their lifestyle to protect their health. They were scared when they had their first attack. But it's even scarier when you realize that almost one out of five men who have that first attack will be dead within a year. What is sad is that their attacks could have been prevented—not only the first attack but the second as well.

The statistics are clear: the odds that you have blockages going on in the arteries throughout your body are overwhelming.

Here are some statistics you want to know:

1. Severe heart attacks resulting in a cardiac arrest often happen with no warning. Now get this stat: only 7.6 percent of people who suffer a complete cardiac arrest *outside* of a hospital setting survive long enough to be discharged. If John watching television in Alaska had waited two more minutes before leaving his house, he would have been one of the 92.4 percent who didn't make it.

2. One-half of individuals who die of sudden cardiac arrest are under the age of sixty-five. Just because you are not in your eighties, don't feel as if you don't need to take care of your arteries. No matter what your age, you need to implement the Prescription for Life plan in your life. Prevent that first attack from happening on any organ in your body.

3. People with high cholesterol counts have about *twice* the risk of heart disease as individuals with lower levels.

Don't be a gambler. Don't even play against the odds. The old saying is, if you're going to be stupid, you've got to be tough. I encourage you to not try to be tough when dealing with the aging process. Don't wait on *symptoms* before deciding to do something smart. And even more important, if you do develop symptoms of an impending heart attack or stroke, and they subside, by all means realize that those symptoms are a flashing red warning light signaling what's going on in your body.

Your goal should be never to have that warning light come on. Your goal should be the *prevention* of any further plaque buildup in your arteries, from this day forth. Halt the process in its tracks now. Prevent your arteries from becoming any older than they are today, and keep them there.

Some things happen to your body that cannot be changed. However, the great majority of what causes the aging process is preventable. Focus on what you can change that will allow you to live longer and younger.

4

Beware of Alternative Ways
to Beat Aging

Let me be as clear as I can be: there are no easy alternatives to defeating the aging process. Developing the proper lifestyle is the only solution. But hardly a day goes by that I don't hear about (or am asked about or read about or see advertised) some type of product that is supposed to make you look or feel younger. Herbal medicines, Asian roots, special juices, and all types of mail-order drugs claim to "enhance" your health in some way.

And when people mention to me how much better they feel after taking such and such, a pill someone sold them on, or some type of herbal medicine or juice to help them lose weight and feel younger, this is the important information I point out to them: herbal medicines and alternative drugs do not undergo the scientific testing that controlled medicines undergo as required by the national Food and Drug Administration.

Let's say you bought a dog who won't obey, and someone comes along and informs you they are selling a special type of bone. If your dog chews on it three times a day, they say, he will start obeying you more. You buy those special bones and begin giving them to your dog. And sure enough, your dog starts obeying you better. Now the question in your mind is, "Did the bone actually help or did the dog simply start obeying me better?" There would be a simple answer to your question if the manufacturer of the special bone had done what is called a *double-blind study*. Such studies are performed by drug companies and reported to the FDA.

The FDA doesn't regulate dog bones, but this is how it would work if they did. The bone manufacturer would get five hundred dogs and give them the special bone. The manufacturer would also get five hundred additional dogs and give them just a regular bone that looks identical to the special bone. The regular one is called a placebo bone. The two bones look alike and taste the same.

Now you mix the two groups together so no one knows who got which bone. Next the manufacturer will get an outside, impartial party to evaluate the thousand dogs and determine which dogs begin to obey much better. This impartial party will be *blind* to which dog got the manufacturer's bone and also *blind* to which dog got the plain placebo bone.

If it is determined that the five hundred who chewed on the special bone actually obeyed better than the five hundred dogs who chewed on the ordinary bone, then the manufacturer's claim is valid. The FDA will give the company permission to sell the bone as advertised. However, if the results of the trial do not show any significant difference between the two groups of dogs, then the "good bone" claim will not be validated by the FDA—and you won't waste your money buying those bones.

Medicines (but not dog bones—sorry) approved by the FDA undergo such double-blind testing. Alternative medicines do not undergo such approved tests, much less pass them.

Your friends have taken such and such a pill and have lost a significant amount of weight. You know them. You believe them. You know what they weighed before they began taking the pill. They swear by it because they have actually taken off pounds. But I have to remind you that personal testimony advertisement is the farthest from the *full* truth you can get.

It was just after spring break at the college when I first saw her. She was sitting on the end of the examining table when I entered the room. She had such a pretty face with a natural smile. She was also a little overweight, but my eyes were immediately drawn to the tips of all her fingers. They were as black as charcoal, and from the base of her fingernails to the tips of her fingers the skin looked like wrinkled, dried black leather. It would look the same if she had gangrene of her fingertips from frostbite.

I held her fingers in my open palm and asked her what had happened. Her only response was, "I don't know." The tips appeared to have no blood flow to the skin, so I felt for a pulse in her wrist. It was pounding strongly. I rubbed the edge of one finger and asked her if she had any sensation—could she feel my rubbing? I was thinking perhaps the problem was neurological, like in leprosy. But she had excellent sensation right down to the necrotic black skin.

I informed her that for some reason the small blood vessels in the tips of her fingers had gone into a prolonged spasm and had cut off the blood supply to her fingertips. I didn't tell her at the time, but I knew she was going to require amputation of the tip of each one of her fingers. She was going to be disfigured for life and lose all tactile ability of touch from her fingertips. She told me the process was beginning to take place in her toes too.

I asked her if she was on any medication. She said for the past four months she had been taking a daily herbal capsule that was supposed to help her lose weight. And she had indeed lost about ten pounds. She related how the capsule had done wonders for several of her friends who had lost considerable weight while taking it.

When she told me she was on some type of herbal medicine, I cringed at what was going through my mind. I knew what she was going to have to go through with the amputations. I recalled how the anesthesiologists at our hospital had complained bitterly about several patients whose blood pressure had dropped insidiously during surgery. The anesthesiologist had to quickly inject medicine intravenously to get their blood pressure back to a normal state—and found out later the patients had been on herbal medicines or alternative medicine pills. These are the ones without the double-blind study and FDA approval.

It also quickly ran through my mind that the anesthesia department at our hospital had such a problem with so many of these alternative medicines that they had accumulated a list of them and made a file of which ones would cause a fall of blood pressure or cause spasm in the lungs when the patient was put to sleep, as well as some that would cause kidney damage after the anesthesia. This young college student had no idea what she was doing and that it had caused those small vessels in her fingertips to spasm. And the sad part was that it was too late to do anything about it. The ends of her fingers were dead.

From a surgical standpoint, removing this young lady's fingertips would not be complicated at all. But for the first time in my surgical career, I realized I did not have the courage it took to perform multiple amputations on this extremely nice young college student. I instructed her to stop taking the medication immediately because there was most likely some ingredient in the medicine that was reacting with the small vessels in the tips of her fingers and toes. I explained I would refer her to a teaching institution, where they could examine the medication and determine exactly what was in it that she was reacting to before they performed the amputations of her fingertips at that hospital.

I would recommend anyone taking herbal medication to discontinue its use—not only the "medicines" for weight loss but also those that are supposed to make you feel better or have more energy or improve your overall health or memory. It may not cause any problem in 99 percent of your friends who are taking it, but you may be the one in a hundred who reacts to the medicine in a permanently damaging way.

Don't be fooled. Personal testimony isn't always a reliable way to evaluate a substance. The college girl with the blackened fingertips is not an isolated case of damage. Until she lost her fingertips, she would have told you the herbal medicine she was taking had helped her lose weight.

Here's another example of the futility of alternative, unapproved treatments. A woman had metastatic cancer that had spread throughout her body. She was presented at the hospital's cancer conference, where all cancer patients were discussed by the medical doctors, the radiation therapists, and the oncologists—the team that decides whether or not to recommend chemotherapy. She had no chance for cure or even palliative extension of her life. The recommendation of the cancer conference doctors was that it would be of no benefit to put her through the perils of the side effects of the medicines and to treat her symptomatically only. This means she would be given some type of pain control medicine to keep her as comfortable as possible for the remaining few months she had left.

However, once informed of the decision, she went to a "doctor" she had been told about who was in another state. Word was that he could treat cancer with some special type of medicine he was getting from somewhere overseas. It was not an FDA approved medication. This "doctor" told her there was a strong chance of curing her cancer. She spent her money and took the treatments, but to no avail. All she received was a false sense of hope.

Whether you want to lose weight or defeat cancer, beware of alternative treatment. If there has not been a certified trial on a drug, if there has not been a double-blind study on the medication, *beware*.

The Prescription for Life plan teaches you how to reach your goal weight safely without taking a single alternative pill to lose an ounce of excess poundage.

5

Prevention Is Key
to Staying Young

Staying as young as possible comes down to one word: *prevention*. So many times a physician prescribes a medicine to *treat* a patient for a problem but does not adequately emphasize what the patient should personally do to fight against the *cause* of the problem. The prevention aspect for good health gets overlooked or minimized. A patient is placed on a certain medication and thinks that is all he or she has to do to keep the arteries clean. This is especially true when someone is placed on a cholesterol-lowering medication. Patients think everything is okay if they take the medicine and their cholesterol numbers are in normal range the next time they have their blood drawn.

According to the National Center for Health Statistics, about one in four Americans over the age of forty-five takes a cholesterol-lowering drug. And the use of statins among people older than forty-five has increased tenfold in the past two decades.

Doctors currently write 255 million prescriptions for cholesterol-lowering drugs each year. Although your doctor should be the one to decide whether you should take such a drug, many without heart disease are taking statins or similar drugs for *preventive* purposes. Some reports have shown, however, a nearly 50 percent increase in diabetes among longtime statin users. There are ways to cut the risks of a heart attack other than medication. Weight loss and exercise are by far safer than taking a pill for the rest of your life.

It is disheartening to hear about patients who have a problem with their cholesterol, or have had surgery on their heart arteries, or have had a stent placed, who think the solution to their problem is a prescribed drug. Prevention may be discussed by the doctor, but somehow the patient doesn't realize prevention is the one thing he or she has control over. Nine out of ten don't even begin changing their lifestyle to prevent the problem from worsening. Most simply take the medicine and continue on with life as they have always lived it.

Not too many months ago a gentleman told me an unbelievable story about a massive heart attack he had two years earlier, when he was in his midfifties. He felt chest pain and was rushed to the hospital in a small town before being air lifted to a city hospital a hundred miles away. He had two blockages in his heart arteries, and doctors immediately attempted to place a stent into each of the blockages. There was some type of complication after the initial stent had been inserted, however, and the remainder of the procedure had to be aborted. The remaining artery was left with a 70 percent blockage. He was already on medication for his blood pressure and was told after the stent was placed that his blood sugar was borderline high and his cholesterol was elevated. He was given medication for his cholesterol and blood pressure.

I asked him what instructions he received about changing his lifestyle after the procedure was completed and he was stable. "I knew I was overweight, and they may have said something about my weight," he told me. He had a sense of excitement in giving me the details he remembered. "But their main focus was on avoiding sodium in my diet. So for the past two years, the main thing my wife and I have constantly focused on has been the amount of salt I eat."

I explained the basis of the Prescription for Life plan to him. (I think it scared him some to hear the truth about where he was heading unless he did something about it.) Then in about a half hour, he committed to a completely new lifestyle. "I want to be around for my children and my future grandchildren," he said. He had a solemn look on his face. Then he began a half smile. "I like the idea that at fifty-five years of age I can completely assure myself that I am not going to end my life with a heart attack."

He finally understood that an alarm had gone off so loudly that he had to do something about his own fate.

He was onboard.

His mind was set.

In follow-up, he had lost most of his excess weight, had developed a completely different style of eating, and was exercising. He now takes a lower dose of his cholesterol medicine, and his blood pressure is in normal range. He is another example of someone who simply did not know what he should be doing. Now that he is informed, he is committed and making a difference he will appreciate the rest of his life.

So whether you are talking about taking extra medication or avoiding sodium, keep in mind the importance of a lifestyle change in addition to your treatment. *Lifestyle change is the key to prevention.*

A False Sense of Security

A pill alone is far from the answer. I remember seeing a scale used to weigh medication to the exact milligram. Two trays were suspended, one on each side of the middle support. The pharmacist would place an exact metal weight on one tray and pour the powdered medication onto the opposite tray until the needle moved exactly to the middle of the scale and both sides were equal.

Some of the things people do thinking they are promoting good health is similar to placing one ounce of truth on one side of the scale and a hundred-pound bag of medical reality on the other. They equate the ounce of prevention they are doing with the hundred pounds of medical significance, things they are not doing. They think their action is in equal proportion to the total overall care of the body. Their ounces consist of eating "lean" beef, "low-fat" cheese, and grass-fed meat, taking daily multivitamins, and the list goes on and on. All of these choices may be "good," but they weigh *ounces* on one side of the scale in comparison to the *pounds* of lifestyle change benefits that are so much more significant to their overall health.

The worst trick you can play on yourself is to believe you are doing something significant to protect your health when at the same time you are doing tenfold harm to your body without realizing it. The basic problem with so many of your "be good to myself" implementations is that you are giving yourself *a false sense of security.* You think you are hunting elephants, but in reality you are only killing gnats.

Numerous people, by their own decision, take an aspirin a day, thinking they are doing something exceedingly important in preventing a heart attack. An aspirin indeed does thin the blood. And if you had those LDL Cholesterol splinters floating around and some got into the wall of your artery and caused your body to respond by declaring battle—and that battle resulted in some bleeding and the wall of that artery burst open and a clot started forming within the lumen of your artery in your heart—aspirin could indeed interfere with the clotting mechanism and prevent that clot from completely plugging off the blood flow in the artery.

The fallacy is that all the while you are taking the aspirin, you are doing nothing for the real basic problem of allowing LDL to enter your arteries. *Aspirin is the hypocrite heart attack preventer.* There should be loudspeakers shouting this reality every time someone takes an aspirin in an effort to prevent a heart attack. The bullhorn should be directed right into the ears of the individual, reminding him or her to prevent the problem in the first place, to not eat the foods that cause LDL to increase, to get to an ideal weight, and to exercise every day.

Nearly a third of middle-aged Americans regularly take a baby aspirin in hopes of preventing a heart attack or stroke. But some doctors report that they are stopping a lot more patients from taking aspirin than they are starting. A recent article in the medical journal *Archives of Internal Medicine* reports on a study of more than one hundred thousand people who had never had a heart attack or stroke. They were given either aspirin or a nonaspirin placebo. Researchers found that the overall risk of dying prematurely is the same with both groups. The aspirin takers are 10 percent less likely to have any type of heart event but were 30 percent more likely to have a serious gastrointestinal bleeding event, a side effect of frequent aspirin use.

In other words, the study concluded that in people without a previous heart attack or stroke, the regular use of aspirin may be more harmful than beneficial. If you haven't had a heart attack or don't have any of the precursors of heart disease, ask your doctor whether or not you should be taking aspirin.

But here's the point in all this. It is my belief that any doctor who instructs you to take aspirin to prevent a clot from forming in the battlefield should also tell you how to *prevent the battle*. If you need to take aspirin, you should definitely establish strategies for preventing a heart attack. If you are not living the proper lifestyle, and only taking the aspirin, you are going bear hunting with a switch. You are giving yourself a false sense of security. If you develop the lifestyle of eating properly to keep your LDL down, exercising to get your HDL up, and eliminating any excess fat from your body that also causes your LDL to be elevated, you are preventing the problem that leads to the clotting to begin with. Focus on preventing the source of the problem.

If your doctor recommends you take an aspirin, by all means take it. But now you also know the importance of developing the proper lifestyle in addition to taking the aspirin.

Don't ever fool yourself into a false sense of security. Even if you are placed on a medicine to lower your cholesterol, or treat your diabetes, or lower your blood pressure, that pill alone is not the complete answer.

I was eating lunch when I received a phone call asking if I could come to a friend's office right then and check his assistant, Mary. She was fifty-eight years old. Three days earlier, her physician had told her she had high cholesterol and gave her a prescription for medication to help bring it down. Twenty-five minutes before I was called, she had taken the first dose of the medicine. Her face quickly flushed with little white splotches, she started breathing rapidly, she became afraid she was going to pass out, and her hands turned red except the tips of her fingers, which blanched as white as snow. Mary was scared. I got in my car and drove the three minutes to her office and examined her. Her pulse was normal, her blood pressure was okay, and everything checked out within normal limits except for the flushing. She had calmed down and was now only upset with her doctor for giving her medicine that scared her to death. I explained that the medication she had just taken occasionally had such side effects. "I will never take it again," was her reply. That opened up an opportunity for me to ask her some practical medical questions.

"Mary, what did your physician instruct you to do in addition to taking the medication to gain control of your cholesterol?" She responded by pulling out the instruction sheet her doctor had given her. It read: "Go on a low-fat diet and take the following medication." That led to my next question: "Do you have the drug company information paper that came with the medicine?"

"I remember a folded paper came with it," she said, "but I didn't read it because it looked too medical for me to understand." She looked at me with a blank stare, her face still flushed.

I explained that the instruction sheet for cholesterol-lowering medicines begins with a statement that such medicine is indicated if—*if*—eating properly, obtaining the proper weight, and exercising have not been successful in getting the cholesterol to a normal range.

Mary's doctor only handed her a piece of paper with two sentences written on it. He didn't stress the need to get her twenty-five excess pounds off. He didn't tell her she needed to join the health club and exercise five days a week. If he had told her to join a club, she would have told him what she told me: she had joined a club almost a year ago. Her definition of exercise consisted of walking their indoor track for twenty minutes at a time. But after the first month, she had not exercised at all—not even the walking.

I told Mary she could get her cholesterol level to normal by controlling what she ate, exercising, and getting her body weight to ideal. I explained what foods she needed to avoid, discussed losing her excess weight, and made her promise to start back at the exercise club beginning that day. Then I asked her to let her doctor know what her plan was and make sure he agreed, which I was certain he would.

I finished by asking Mary a simple question: "Will you commit to begin this new lifestyle to control your health?" I asked her that straight out because I knew she was the type who would honor a commitment to herself. Mary assured me she would.

But prevention won't happen if there is no commitment.

6

Commitment and Action
Are Key to Success

If staying as young as possible comes down to prevention, prevention comes down to one word: *commitment*.

I see it everywhere—with the young, the old, the rich, the poor. And I have to ask myself, Why? Why are they so complacent? So unworried? I watch what they are eating. I see how they are moving around and how they look. I see their weight. The picture I perceive is a snake that makes no noise until it strikes. These people will remain complacent until a symptom occurs. And then they just accept it as the natural process of aging.

I want to help them. I want to offer answers that will make a difference. And I know their problem. They do not have the commitment to do what is necessary to defeat the enemy of aging. They've made the *decision* numerous times before but don't add the *commitment*. They do some "ounce" prevention, like multivitamins or an aspirin every day. Some even brag about eating free-range beef. But they never take the action required for success.

I want you to be different. If you'll make an effort to realize the following truths, you'll experience success in reaching a point of commitment. See where you are in the process, then commit to working toward success in the plan.

1. Realize the *Need*

Few realize the need. So many who are overweight or don't exercise, who are eating themselves into the grave, who are developing dementia, high blood pressure, or diabetes never see the need to eat properly, to get to an ideal weight, or to exercise. They are given a pill to get their cholesterol down, a pill to lower their blood pressure, another pill to control their sugar, and they take an aspirin to prevent a heart attack. They simply do not see the need to do more. But a pill isn't enough. So many do not realize that being treated with pills is not the same kind of protection prevention is. There is so much you can personally do to prevent your problem. Work at it—you may be able to eliminate having to take the pill. (Or at least get the dose lower.)

2. Many *Want* to . . . But

Many actually do realize the need and want to make their lives better. They want to lose weight. They really want to be more active. Deep in their hearts, they want to—but don't. Life is too hard. They have to deal with too many other things first: their job, their marriage, their children. Or they're just too busy to do anything right now. Many want to—but later, not right now. The trouble is, later may never come.

3. *Decision* Is a Change of Mind

This is the tough one. Many want to have *moments* when they decide to do something about their health. Many New Year's resolutions to lose weight are made in all sincerity. Some of these people read about what is causing their problems. Or even better, they learn what they can do to prevent the aging process from developing so fast. They actually hear that the LDL Cholesterol is the bad one that causes some kind of problem with their arteries. They develop some kind of an understanding that the HDL Cholesterol is the hero and that exercise will increase those particles. And that weight loss does the same. They decide to lose weight. Some even study the benefits of getting to an ideal weight. They *decide* they are going to change their eating habits. They *decide* no more red meat, no more egg yolks, no more cheese or whole milk. They *decide* to cut out the butter and margarine. They *decide* to set up an exercise program and to maintain an ideal weight.

The problem is that a decision does not require action. A decision is simply a change of mind. Decision is an essential first step, but so many times, it stops there. These are the ones who have had a stent placed or have been told for the first time they are diabetic or have high blood pressure. Or they are the ones who feel perfectly healthy and have been told how to prevent future problems. If they have the knowledge, many decide to do something about their problem—but they fail when the time for action arrives.

4. *Commitment* Is a Change of Heart

One day it came to me. Immediate action is the most significant point required for success. All the knowledge in the world isn't going to prevent your aging process unless you come to this realization. Even if you read this book three times and learn all the medical aspects of aging, you won't do anything about it without this insight. It is called commitment.

Proverbs 23:7 states that as a man "thinketh in his heart, so is he." That is so true. Your "wants" have to go deeper than just in your mind. They have to reach your heart.

Commitment requires a change of heart—it requires action. *Decision involves the mind—commitment involves the heart.* We've covered the basics of the causes of aging. You now understand that the most significant aspect of aging is directly related to protecting your arteries. You understand completely the damage within the walls of your arteries whenever an LDL Cholesterol splinter enters the media. And most important, you have come to realize that saturated fat in the foods you eat causes the greatest increase in your LDL Cholesterol. You have the basic knowledge, you have made the commitment, and now your success depends on your actions.

Case Studies on Commitment

Susie

Susie is sixty-one years old. She has had an active life, traveled the world over, and is financially well off. She went for her annual checkup, and her doctor informed her she had developed diabetes. Even though it was mild, it required medication. She was worried that her new diagnosis would lead to health problems as time went on. I showed her a medical report I recently read. It pointed out that being told you have diabetes has the same outcome as being told you just survived your first heart attack. She was shocked to find out that diabetes is as serious as having a heart attack. I pointed out that the American Diabetes Association says that 8.3 percent of the population has diabetes and that heart disease is the number one killer of diabetic people. I explained that she is not alone; one in five has some elevation of their blood sugar.

But what affected Susie the most was when I explained that if she didn't take action to control her diabetes she would most likely die of a heart attack. As she wiped the tears off her cheeks, she told me she had no idea diabetes was that serious. I talked to her earnestly, explaining how she could get her blood sugar down to normal and be able to come off her medication. All it was going to take was losing her extra pounds, getting an exercise program going, and eating the proper foods. It was fairly simple.

The first week, she began walking daily and changing her eating habits. She was feeling good. And I remember feeling so happy that she had *decided* to change her lifestyle. After that first week, my wife and I invited her to go out to dinner. I wanted to see what she would order for her meal. She didn't eat the premeal bread. She ordered a salad and a fat-free dressing—on the side. Her main course was grilled fish. I was feeling good that my two-hour dissertation had taken proper effect.

However, when we were leaving the restaurant, she and my wife walked out ahead of me as I stopped to speak to someone I knew. On the way out, there was a little bowl of wrapped mints. Susie didn't see me watching, but my eyes followed her fingers as she picked up two of the mints and slid them into her purse. Not one, but two.

I realized Susie had *decided* to change her lifestyle to gain control of her diabetes, but she had not made the *commitment.* Taking the two mints was a very small thing, but it made me afraid that Susie would stay on medication for diabetes the rest of her life. Because of her little decision to take the mints, she would have difficulty accomplishing the big things necessary to control her diabetes. She will have difficulty controlling her future because she didn't take control of her present. My hope is that she doesn't have to go on insulin as she gets older, and that she will revamp her thinking and commit to a new lifestyle.

Many times you will hit a little thing that will trip you. That doesn't mean you are going to lose the football game, but it does mean you have to reevaluate your decision and commitment. It means you have stumbled and need to get right back up and get going again.

By the way, Susie found hope in one particular article. According to the Centers for Disease Control, type 2 diabetes accounts for 90 to 95 percent of all diabetes cases and can be prevented through lifestyle changes. But by losing approximately 7 percent of body weight, along with improving diet and exercising, it is very likely people can prevent diabetes from ever developing. And if you are diabetic like Susie, the same lifestyle may even return your glucose levels to normal.

It has been two years since I had my two-hour dissertation with Susie concerning her diabetes. My wife and I took her out to eat recently. She had made the *decision* to change her lifestyle of eating, exercising, and getting to her ideal weight, but I was concerned that she had not made the *commitment.* She has gained a little weight. Her exercise program lasted only about three weeks. Her eating habits haven't changed significantly—although, she didn't order anything fried. She is still on medication for her diabetes.

I told her about watching her take two mints as she left the restaurant that night. She just laughed and then, almost boastingly, told me, "Most of the time I now take only a single mint as I leave." (She didn't want to sound completely defeated.)

Susie will most likely die from a heart attack years before she has to. Looking back, I wish I had asked her to sign a commitment pledge concerning her *decision* to beat diabetes. I wish I had explained to her the difference between making a decision to change her lifestyle of eating, exercising, and weight loss and making a *commitment* to do so. I wish I had explained to her in a little more detail that the small things she would do wrong would be red flag warnings for her to get back on course. I wish I had taken the time to encourage her not simply to decide in her mind that she was going to defeat diabetes but also to commit in her heart to take the action necessary to be successful.

But I didn't. Susie made the decision but not the commitment. She can change, and I hope she does. But commitment is the key.

J. B.

J. B. was near 350 pounds when I first met him. That was about ten years ago. He was the strongest man I had ever personally met. He could lift more weight than most any football player. His arms were bigger around than my thighs. He had the muscle, but he also had the fat. Over the years, the fat kept increasing until he reached his obesity weight. That was his condition when I saw him about a year ago.

I ran into him the other day. He was much trimmer. He had lost over sixty pounds, and he was smiling when he reached out his hand to shake mine. He told me his story.

He had reached the point where his doctor informed him that if he didn't lose weight he was going to die. "I didn't like that statement," J. B. said. "The doctor told me to go to a certain nearby retirement village. This was one where you start out in a cottage, and as your health worsens, you move into a rest home, and later, when you are bedridden, they move you into the nursing home part. My doctor told me when I left his office that I wouldn't find any fat people at the nursing home—because they were all dead." J. B. looked at me with his hands turned upward and told me that he did go look. "And there were no fat people there. They had already died," he said.

That was his moment of *commitment*. He made the *decision* that day to lose his excess weight. He said he was going to lose another forty pounds. He asked me to go over a plan for him, and that was how we spent the next hour. What he had been doing had worked for losing weight, but he had not developed a plan for what to do when he reached his goal weight. The first part of our discussion centered on his ideal weight. He had been in his best shape at 195 pounds when he began college. He realized he could reach that again if he set it as his ideal weight goal. Then we discussed the importance of developing a lifestyle of eating now that he can continue once he reaches his ideal weight. He was so thankful for all the information.

Two hours later, I received a phone call from him asking some specifics about his elevated cholesterol. He wants knowledge. He has done well on his own without a specific plan. But now, J. B. sees himself as successful—because he is *committed*.

Knowledge is essential but can be void without commitment. The worst heartbreak I have seen a person experience is when they have had a major setback health-wise and realize they should have been taking better care of themselves. They understand then that what they now want they can never have. Their lifestyle has left them with permanent damage. What they have sown they are now reaping. I encourage you not to travel that road. Work on your future—beginning today.

I know you have made the *decision* to improve your health. Right now I want you to *commit* to developing three strategies for your new lifestyle. The first is to eat healthy. That means you will commit to not eating specific foods that damage the arteries in your body, as well as pledging to yourself to eat specific foods that protect your body. The second commitment is to control your weight, to reach and maintain what you determine is your ideal weight. And the third commitment is to develop a personal exercise program.

These are the three strategies that will determine your physiological age. These are the three strategies that will become routine habits that control the aging process of your body. Don't

COMMITMENT FORM

My Commitment Statement

_____

_____

_____

_____

_____

_____

Signed   Date wait for a crisis. Commit now to do everything in your power to develop a younger, more active and productive body and mind.

Many decide.

Few commit.

By the way, you remember Mary from the last chapter, the fifty-eight-year-old woman who had taken some medication for her cholesterol? Her face had flushed, she had begun breathing rapidly, and her hands had turned red except the tips of her fingers, which had blanched white. Well, I saw her two months after she had made the *commitment* to change her lifestyle. She had lost over sixteen pounds and told me she had changed her eating habits completely. She is exercising five days a week.

She has acknowledged to herself that her warning light had come on, and she was frightened by a great wake-up call. The episode she experienced was the best caution light she has ever seen, because that attack resulted in commitment to take care of her health. It took the medicine reaction to scare her enough to change her lifestyle to eating properly, losing weight, and exercising for the rest of her life. It exposed her false sense of security in depending on a pill alone.

How to Get from Here to There

It's one thing to change your mind and heart, and it is another to get going.

The Little Things Count

Football legend Vince Lombardi, who coached the Green Bay Packers for nine years, had the best winning percentage of any National Football League coach with at least eighty-five victories. Attention to detail made him a winner. He didn't want his players to be merely good; he insisted they strive to be the best. And he summed it all up when he stated he was convinced that it was the small things that won football games.

Get that, *the small things won the game.* Oh sure, he had to have a man who could run the ball up the middle like a house afire, and he had to have someone who could throw the ball like a rocket and another player who could catch anything that hit his fingertips. Those were the big things in the game. But what made those players get that way was how they handled the little things. Little things, like the receiver who stayed after practice and caught ball after ball; the quarterback who took his playbook home and studied and studied his responsibility in each play while everyone else was relaxing for the night; the lineman who knew exactly where he was going to place his left foot when he lined up to play because he had practiced moving that foot back about a half-inch, assuring himself that he was developing the added power to beat his opponent.

Lombardi makes you realize it is the little things in life that make the biggest outcomes possible. Commitment begins with attention to the little things that reassure you that the big thing is going to happen.

I remember hearing about J. C. Penney when he opened his first department store. At his five o'clock closing time, he would walk outside the front door of the store to see if anyone was coming down the sidewalk. If there was no one in sight, he would go back inside, lock the door, and close for the day. But if he saw someone coming, he would wait to see if they might be coming to the store. He never wanted to miss a potential sale. That attitude every day at closing time was a small part of the overall success of his business, but the little things, so many times, determine how the big things turn out.

Small things you do will let you know whether or not you are going to succeed; they forecast your future. Small signs will signal whether or not you are persistent. Tiny red flags will wave from time to time, and you must condition yourself to watch for them. And at that *moment*, you must make that extra little effort to take care of the little things.

Then when your commitment is solid, you will begin to notice little changes you are doing differently. For instance, you've set a specific time to exercise daily rather than "maybe sometime today." You've determined your menu for the day: what you will eat and what you won't dare eat. You've decided in advance not to eat that second helping of whatever. You've gotten specific with your plan. You have begun action on the small things that will win the game for you.

The Ten-Minute Factor

He was about fifty years old and had smoked most of his life. It was usually just a pack a day, but he admitted to a couple of packs some days on the weekend—especially when he went fishing. I knew he was left-handed, in what hand he held his cigarettes, because of the nicotine stain between two of the fingers on his left hand.

I was seeing him for his final follow-up after I had worked him up for a possible cancer in his lung. He didn't have any insurance but told me, "I will pay you a little every month." The tumor had turned out not to be malignant, but I explained that if he continued smoking, a cancerous tumor could develop in his lung. I used the example of him standing in the middle of the road in front of my office and seeing a tractor-trailer truck coming down the hill. I asked him if he would get out of the road or just stand there and let it run over him. (He made his living driving tractor-trailers.) He stated he would get out of the road.

I then informed him his cigarettes were that truck, and if he didn't quit smoking, he would eventually get run over. I told him about the ten-minute factor, explaining that everyone can control their addiction for a ten-minute period and that he could quit smoking if he would apply that little secret to his own smoking habits. "Whenever you get the urge to smoke," I said, "just tell yourself you are not going to do it for the next ten minutes. Then get to doing something else. Whenever the urge hits you again, do the same thing." That's about all I told him, not expecting him to do it, especially on Saturdays.

I want to introduce you to this dynamic secret too. It not only works for quitting smoking but also allows you to be successful in controlling your weight and your eating habits. This trick makes it possible for you not to snack on that piece of chocolate or not to order that steak. It will enable you to make a salad with fruit on it. It is the most important and amazing self-control tool I know. It is the spark that makes things happen, the spark that gives you hope.

I know individuals who have controlled their addiction to harmful foods by using this method. I know people who have never smoked another cigarette after adopting this process. And you can control what you eat by using this same principle. It is the motivating force for learning self-control. It is one of the foundations of forming habits. Use this factor once, and then a second and third time, and before long, a habit is ingrained into your mind.

It is called the *ten-minute factor*. It is a dynamic component of reasoning that doesn't suggest what you can do—it demands it (at least for a period of ten minutes). I first heard of it when I was in Alaska, fishing with a man in his sixties who had at one time been addicted to drugs as well as to cigarettes. As he was showing me one of his favorite fishing sites on the backside of a cove of a large lake, he told me his story.

He had been in prison because he couldn't control his habits. One day he realized that he couldn't control them for the rest of his life—*but he could control them for ten minutes.* He tried this concept with his smoking. Whenever he had an urge to smoke, he would simply tell himself he wasn't quitting smoking for good, that he would allow himself a cigarette later on that day, but for the next ten minutes, he was in charge—and he was not going to smoke.

He would then get busy doing something else and not light up. He would go outside and work on something, or get a cup of coffee, or start reading, or turn on the television. He said the urge to smoke would return in an hour or so, and he would trigger his *ten-minute factor* again. He pointed out that since implementing the ten-minute factor over twenty years ago he had never smoked another cigarette. He said it worked the same way with alcohol and drugs. He was motivated to change his lifestyle, and he committed to it, ten minutes at a time.

That story impressed me so much that I began applying his strategy to the wrong foods I had a craving for. I began sharing it with others who had made the decision to change their lifestyle of eating, as well as of weight control and exercise. I shared it with my patients who had lung disease and smoked. The *ten-minute factor* secret has worked time and again with the addiction of smoking. It has worked on drug addiction and alcohol addiction.

The reason it is so important for success in the Prescription for Life plan is that you are addicted to the foods you eat. An addiction is the end result of habit. Before someone gets addicted to smoking or alcohol, they develop a habit of smoking or drinking. You become addicted to chocolate or cheese or any other foods that really taste good simply because you develop a habit of eating these foods, develop a desire for their taste, and then continue eating them on a regular basis. Poor eating habits turn into eating addictions.

You are going to learn how to begin working on avoiding certain foods you may be addicted to. The same way bad eating habits lead to an addiction, good eating habits help you develop a good eating lifestyle.

At some point you are going to have to make a decision. It is so important, because it could change your life in so many different aspects. Don't take the *ten-minute factor* lightly. You don't want to be one of those who keep sitting on a fence, simply thinking about losing weight, or developing the proper eating habits, or starting to exercise (someday). This is a tool that will allow you to do something about developing your lifestyle. To decide today to exercise, to lose weight, or to stop eating the wrong foods is a process. It takes about two months to be able to substitute one good food for a harmful one. The nice part is that down the road you will enjoy the new, healthy food the way you enjoyed the old, damaging one. The day will come when you could not care less about eating a bite of a food that is so dear to you today. In fact, you will look back and believe that food was not all that good to begin with.

Smoking is the worst addiction to overcome. We can learn by looking at the worst. I know there are advertisements about patches and pills that make you "cut down" on the desire to smoke. I have operated on numerous patients who were addicted to smoking. I have had some patients beat the addiction and many who could not. True knowledge comes from learning how the ones who quit did so. But I have never had a patient who cut down on smoking and then was able to quit permanently.

I recall an instructor I had when I was rotating through orthopedics in my surgical training. He very proudly announced to all of us medical students that he was on a program to beat his addiction to smoking. He even announced the date it would happen. It was about three months down the road. He smoked fewer and fewer cigarettes per day, checking off the daily time chart he was following. He slowed down, day by day, and finally the last day of the plan arrived. We all gathered in the doctor's lounge to watch him smoke his last cigarette.

He smiled and gave an upward glance of sureness as he tapped a cigarette out of the pack and tossed the remaining cigarettes into the wastebasket. He stretched out both arms as he held his cigarette lighter in his left hand and the lone survivor cigarette in his right. As he brought both hands toward his mouth, he announced, very distinctly, "My last one," and lit it up. We all smiled and clapped as he took a long drag and inhaled. I will never forget how he smashed the cigarette butt in the ashtray as he looked around the room, smiling at each of us only as one could in complete victory.

His cessation of smoking lasted a total of three days before he lit up again. His immediate reason for failure? *Desire.* He said, almost sadly, that his desire for smoking was still there. He had tapered down to one cigarette per day, but tapering hadn't overcome the desire.

Moderation won't beat desire. Moderation can get you killed.

He taught me a lesson about controlling smoking, or eating the wrong foods, or beating any other addiction. You have to gain control over the desire, or you will never beat the addiction. And to beat the desire, don't taper. Abstain.

If you acknowledge your addiction to foods like cookies and ice cream and donuts and candy, cheese, red meats, and multiple fried foods, you can overcome that addiction. It won't be by slowing down, day by day, in hopes that on a certain day in the future you won't have any desire for that particular food. Abstain completely from it for a two-month period, ten minutes at a time. Not just eating less and less of it for two months, believing the desire won't be there three days later. You abstain completely while developing new habit foods to build your new eating lifestyle.

Let me point out the key to beating the addiction of certain lethal foods you like: get rid of the bad stuff in your home. Do you think it would be smart for someone who is addicted to alcohol to keep a fifth of Jack Daniels in his cupboard? Should he have it just in case his willpower broke one day? I don't think so. Why have something that is going to be a constant temptation nearby?

It's the same thing with harmful foods. Let's say you get ready for bed, walk through the kitchen, and all of a sudden you have the desire for a piece of chocolate. You know exactly where you keep some. Odds are you will go to your hiding place and pull out a piece and eat it. After all, you deserve it because you ran three miles that day, didn't eat a single piece of bread at the restaurant where you had dinner, and haven't eaten any dessert in over a week. However, if there is no chocolate in the house, this time you'll simply go on back to your bedroom.

Beating the addiction to foods begins at home. Commit to not having any of your addictive foods in your household. Get rid of the foods containing the "bad threes": saturated fat, trans fat, and cholesterol. Get rid of the bad cooking oil. Switch out your butter for a substitute that has zero saturated fat, zero trans fat, and zero cholesterol. Have skim milk rather than either 2 percent or whole milk in your refrigerator. Get rid of your high saturated fat cookies and cakes and processed foods. Throw out the cheese. Toss out any chips that aren't zero, zero, zero.

Breaking down any unhealthy eating addictions you may have and laying the foundation for good eating habits take only ten minutes at a time.

A Ten-Minute Success Story

I was seeing patients in my office one afternoon when my nurse told me a gentleman wanted to see me. He didn't have an appointment but wanted just a minute to talk in the hallway.

I looked up the hallway toward the lobby and saw him. He had on tan Carhartt pants, covering a pair of well-worn work boots. The rim of his baseball cap was also well-worn, especially at the left front corner of the bill. His smile was as big as his extended hand, held out to me as I walked up the hall.

As he shook my hand, he said, "It's been exactly one year."

I wasn't sure what in the world he was talking about, but he continued.

"It's been a year since I walked out of your office. When I got in my truck, I pulled the pack of cigarettes out of my pocket and laid them on my dash. They stayed there for the next two months. I wanted to prove to myself that I could beat the habit. Every day, I would look at those cigarettes and shake my head. Ten minutes was all it took. Every time I wanted one, I wouldn't smoke it for ten minutes, just like you said. Finally, I didn't even want one anymore, and I threw them away. And as of today, I haven't smoked in a year, and I just wanted to let you know. I got out of the way of that truck you talked about coming down the road."

I started to congratulate him, but he was already walking back up the hallway, past the nurse and another patient. It took him only a *moment* exactly a year ago in the examining room to make his decision and only ten minutes at a time to make it happen. I am glad he wanted me to know. He will never understand how it pleased me to know he had made a commitment because of what I said.

This patient was told how to improve his lifestyle, and he did something about it. You can do the same. This is when you will link your blood lipid profile to your arteries. This is when you begin to understand that what you eat directly affects your arteries.

Habits: How to Autopilot Life

Over 95 percent of what we do, we do out of habit. Every night when you go to bed, you get in on the same side. You don't stop to think which side of the bed you sleep on or which side your spouse is going to end up on tonight. No, out of habit, you simply get into bed and go to sleep. Some habits are easy to change, but most are difficult.

Habits are important to develop properly because they are the foundation to consistent behavior.

I am a pilot, and I have flown the narrow airway across Cuba at twenty-eight hundred feet. I have flown a smaller aircraft up the Alaskan highway at eight hundred feet. I have flown through gorgeous weather as well as through storms. At times, so many things that require your full concentration are happening that you need all the help you can get. Bad weather is one of the signals that tells me to throw on the autopilot switch. The autopilot is a big help. You simply set the course, and it aids in holding the line.

Habits become your lifestyle autopilot. Develop the right habits related to exercise, the foods you eat, and weight control, and then turn on your autopilot. What once was a challenging decision as to whether you are going to eat a certain food becomes no decision at all. There is no decision to be made about exercising, because you are going to exercise today. Once you stand on the scale and see that you are a pound over your goal weight, you don't have to decide there will be no snacks today and that your meal portions are going to be smaller. At that point, your habits come into play and you will do ten things automatically because your mind goes on autopilot once you step off the scale. Your habits eventually become your lifestyle autopilot, and flying through the day becomes so much easier.

Use the ten-minute factor to help develop your habits. Small steps set up big changes in your life. Develop habits that protect you before the event happens. Decide before you go into a restaurant that you are not going to eat the bread before the meal—such calories are completely superfluous. Eating x number of calories of bread before your entrée does not mean you are going to eat x number fewer calories of your main meal. Decide before you go into a restaurant that you are not going to pick up two or three mints from a tray when you exit. The next time you are already at your goal weight and allow yourself to eat a snack, use the ten-minute factor to eat fruit or nuts this time.

Sooner than you think, you will have formed habits that require no instant decision making. With developing your habits, you will build hope and optimism that you are going to be successful in developing your ideal lifestyle. You will begin seeing yourself younger today. The Prescription for Life plan gives new light to a dark picture.

Setting Goals

A person's goal is everything. The higher the goal, the more the success in what you are attempting. Because your most prized possession is your health, make it your goal to succeed in your Prescription for Life plan.

Setting your goal is the single most essential thing in losing your excess weight. Without a goal, you can't make it happen. You can memorize all the secrets concerning losing weight, but it won't happen unless you set a goal. Reaching a goal requires both decision and commitment. A decision alone won't get you there. Without the self-commitment, it will be a battle for naught. The other side of the coin is just as simple: if you set your goal weight and commit to it, you will reach that ideal weight.

Researchers at the Rush University Medical Center in Chicago interviewed more than twelve hundred elder adults and found something interesting concerning setting goals. They aren't certain why, but their study found that the individuals who had goals were about half as likely to die over a five-year follow-up as those who didn't have definite plans for their future.

If *yesterday* you had a life-debilitating heart attack or began developing dementia caused from the blockage of your arteries to your brain, I guarantee you that *today* I could sell this plan to you. And you would do everything possible to get your hands on whatever amount of money you needed to buy it.

I only ask you to be true to yourself. How do you want to live out the rest of your life? How do you want to live out this next year? And probably the most important question is, How do you want to live out the rest of today?

The purpose of the Prescription for Life plan is not to give you a list of black-and-white do's and don'ts. It is to inform you so that you can make your own decisions about the direction you are going to take. Your goals will decide the quality of the rest of your days here on earth.

I am big into setting goals. As a matter of fact, shortly after completing my surgical training, I wrote a book on goal setting.

Ninety-two percent of people never set a goal. They have "want-to-be," "would-like-to-be," and "wish" lists, but they never get around to actually deciding on a goal for their lives. Ninety-two percent.

And on top of that, only a fraction of the ones who do set goals ever write them down. There is something almost magical about writing your goals down on paper. That is what I would like you to do today. Set your goals to develop the very best lifestyle possible as an individual, and write them down. (Even if it's on a napkin, write them down.)

After you get them on paper, carry them with you in your wallet or purse. Post them in places where you can review them daily. Stick them on your bathroom mirror. Renew your commitment to achieve your goals daily. By the end of this book, you will have written specific goals concerning foods you will eat as well as foods you will never taste again. You will have specific goals for your exercise. You will have a goal weight set in stone, and after you achieve your ideal weight, you will stick to that weight.

You will be specific about your lifestyle. It will be yours and yours alone. Your plan will not be exactly like anyone else's; you will fine-tune it to your personality, your body build, what you do in your life. It won't be one size fits all; it will be customized for you.

You begin by setting *major goals* about each of your three strategies. These will be the goals you set for how you want to end up. You will set up a major goal concerning your eating habits, your weight, and your exercise schedule. You will determine the major goal of what you want your lifestyle to be a year from now, two years from now.

As we go further, you will break those major goals down into *intermediate goals*. These intermediate goals will be more specific and to the point. These intermediate goals will give you the details of what you are going to have to do to accomplish your major goals. These are the "by such-and-such-a-date" goals.

Finally, and most important, will be your *immediate action goals*. These will be goals for what you will do today to set the foundation on which you will build your major lifestyle. These immediate action goals will be the ones that require action today. These are the goals you must reach before going to bed tonight. The reason I say the immediate action goals are the most important ones you will set is because in the overall structure of goal setting, your *immediate action* goals tell you by the end of the day whether or not you are going to reach your major goals. These are the kinds of goals that would have kept Susie from reaching into the bowl of mints on the way out of the restaurant that evening.

If you don't act on your immediate action goals, you will never reach your major goals. Your mind receives a reward each time you accomplish an immediate action goal. The reward is knowing that you are on track in achieving your major goals. Immediate action goals let you know your plan is going to work. They give you true hope. They are the kinds of goals Lombardi would have been talking about when he emphasized the small things making the biggest difference in reaching victory.

Setting goals results in positive emotions. They teach you to believe in yourself when everyone else questions your future success. Here is how it works.

Let's say you need something to motivate you to change your eating habits. You need motivation to lose weight and to have an exercise routine that is similar to going to work every day. Set a major goal on paper. Begin organizing your changes in life that will be required to reach that major goal. Set a specific time to exercise. You have your ideal goal weight nailed down. You have a list of foods you are not going to eat. You have written down the majority of everyday meals you are going to consume. By getting the specifics written, you have the intermediate goal system in order.

Now comes the motivating part of the system. With the immediate action goals you are going to accomplish right now, today, you are going to feel *immediate success* and accomplishment with each immediate action you do. With every immediate action goal you accomplish, you are going to begin seeing yourself already eating the proper foods, already weighing that ideal weight, and already completing the exercise routine you are striving for. With each immediate action goal accomplished, you are chipping away on the major goal and will grasp the realization that you are capable of developing the healthy lifestyle you desire. The immediate action part is your motivator. It is the key to your hope and optimism.

Your positive mind-set will build day by day as you progress through each immediate action goal for each day. To reach your full potential, to reach your major goal of being as young as possible, you must succeed in your immediate action goals. Those actions generate the hope that little alterations lead to big changes. You will have victory in not eating that dessert, passing up the afternoon chocolate chip cookie, and applying the ten-minute factor. Those small victories show you that the big can happen. As you achieve each immediate action goal, you realize you can succeed. You develop the habit of winning.

Nothing's free in life. This plan will mean doing some things you don't like to do. Become a member of the elite 8 percent who set goals. Set your major, intermediate, and immediate action goals. Write them down and concentrate on them—today. The Prescription for Life plan will show you how to achieve them.

Accountability

And last, make yourself accountable to someone. It may be your spouse or a friend who has also realized the necessity of changing their lifestyle. Or it may be a group that wants the encouragement from others who are on the same pathway.

Peer pressure works in mysterious ways. Get with a partner or group to develop your habits together. Organize your own group. Get with individuals at work to make the commitment. Get a group at your church to join you. Or friends from another group you meet with on a routine basis. Communicate daily. Encourage one another. Reinforce the good and underline the bad for each other. Exercise together. Set a time to go to the gym. Ask others what they had for lunch. Accountability and teamwork go hand in hand. A recent study shows that participants with an accountability partner lost 20 percent more weight than individuals who were also losing weight but did not have accountability partners.

Part 2

Eat the Right Foods

My initial awakening to the realization that I needed to do something differently in my lifestyle came when I realized I had increased the waist size of my trousers for the third time in three years. My first moment of decision about changing my lifestyle to improve my overall health came when I realized I needed to lose weight. As time went on, I saw the significance of exercise in getting my heart as strong as possible. After that point, I thought I was doing everything needed to be in good shape. I did not realize that attacking the aging process was a lot more than just getting in good physical shape and trimming down.

It was only after I began reading specific articles in the medical literature concerning the damaging foods I was routinely eating that I realized I was missing out on one of the most significant of the three lifestyle changes I needed.

I realized that eating the right foods was the cornerstone of our plan.

I had read about marathon runners who were trim and very active but who died of a heart attack in the middle of the run. I had heard about people in their forties who appeared healthy but suddenly had a heart attack with no warning at all. I was operating on arteries in patients who were not obese, who played golf and tennis frequently, who I would have agreed were doing what they should to beat the aging process. Yet they would have plaque buildup in their arteries. I sewed bypass grafts around these blockages but never realized I needed to tell the patients what foods to never eat again to keep more plaque from forming.

Finally, it occurred to me that the foods they were eating were the culprits. Even though many patients were doing two of the three parts of the Prescription for Life plan, they were leaving out a crucial segment that was nullifying the other two.

All three strategies are tightly knit together, but I am going to present them in a different order than I came across them because I feel eating the right food is the place to start. It is essential to conquer this one from the get-go. Once you understand how the food strategy works, you will see how it and ideal weight and exercise all intertwine to reward you with that great gift of good health.

7

Food Lessons
from around the World

I have been to many third world hospitals and have operated on people from many nationalities whose diets are different from most typical eating habits in America. Those experiences have taught me a great lesson I will pass on to you.

First of all, I noticed a marked difference in the type of operations I was performing. Back home, many of my procedures were on blocked arteries. I would open carotid arteries leading to the brain that were 85 to 95 percent blocked by plaque buildup, would clean out the plaque, and would close the opening I had made in the artery to do my work. On other patients, I would bypass complete blockages in the arteries going to the legs. I saw patients needing stents and bypass surgery on arteries in their hearts. In the United States, everywhere I looked, I found plaque.

But in the remote areas of Africa, it was different. I will never forget performing an abdominal operation on an elderly man. He had extremely curly gray hair, and the skin around his eyes and mouth were wrinkled from his constant smile. He was thin. His wife was equally thin. (She also had a round piece of carved wood, the size of a quarter, in each ear lobe.) I say they were elderly because they, like most of the elderly in that village, didn't know exactly what year they were born. All I can say is that he had to be in his mideighties.

Once I began operating, I felt for his aorta, the largest artery in the abdomen. It was smooth as silk and so soft, I could hardly believe it.

I felt further for his smaller arteries—and found the same thing.

I felt for the small artery that feeds the small intestines, the artery that got my father. It was as soft and plaque-free as a newborn's.

I operated on another elderly African gentleman whose main artery to his leg felt as soft and pliable as a ten-year-old boy's vessel.

In all the years I operated there, I never operated on an artery that was plugged with plaque. I never saw a patient who needed a stent placed into their heart arteries—or a bypass operation.

What makes their arteries so much different from those of the patients in America? Is it where they live? Is it their race or tribe? Or could it be what foods they *don't* eat?

I had the same experience when I went to Papua New Guinea years ago. I had been told that was where the most primitive group of people on earth lived. When I got there, I could believe it. They wore very little clothing, and none of it was made out of cloth. They used bark and vines and tiny strips of leaves to weave their clothes. The only thing the women wore was a simple skirt around their waist, and the men wore even less. The women carried their small children in a woven net on their backs everywhere they went. I never heard any of the babies crying. The men wore a hollow gourd about twelve inches long and as big around as a circle you make by placing your index finger tip to the tip of your thumb. The gourd was placed over the penis with the tip of the gourd being held by a simple string running from the gourd to around their waist. (It didn't look very comfortable when they ran.)

They were all thin. I could not find an ounce of fat anywhere on their bodies. Neither could I find four medical problems that I searched for. I saw no heart attacks, no strokes, and no disease resulting from arterial damage. Plus, I saw no colon cancer and no breast cancer. Now, those were just observations of a young surgeon on a trip evaluating village after village to see if there was a need for volunteer physicians to come help them. I didn't really understand why there were no medical problems like we see here in developed countries. At the time, I didn't realize that they carried a lesson for us here at home that could prevent coronary artery disease and strokes and even help in preventing certain cancers, especially colon and breast.

But I did see that 99 percent of their food was a sweet potato type of root. Vegetarians here in the States don't know what vegetarian really means unless they have been to those primitive tribes.

It wasn't until years later that I began reading about these people in New Guinea and certain areas of Africa. I read studies in the medical literature about how these tribal people had been evaluated for their cholesterol numbers. Their Total Cholesterol averaged around 150. At that level, almost no heart attacks ever happen. Arteries of such people are going to stay physiologically young for years and years. It was intriguing to realize that the two main sources of harmful foods in America were not available in these tribal areas. They didn't have animal-based foods or dairy products. They didn't have red meat and cheese.

It was a strange feeling to begin understanding what I had seen as a younger surgeon. I started realizing that what protected those primitive people was their diet. It was also a strange feeling to realize that more than half of Americans are dying because of what we are eating.

The tribal people in New Guinea don't have our problems related to the arteries of our hearts and brains because they don't eat the foods that damage those arteries. They don't load their bodies with lethal LDL Cholesterol. I became more interested and began studying more articles about other parts of the world where mainly vegetables and fruits are eaten, with basically no meats or dairy products such as cheese or butter or cream. I began to understand why I didn't see any colon cancer and very little breast cancer in those parts of the world. However, if you moved a thousand of those people to this country and they began eating like most do and gaining weight and sitting around all day, you'd begin seeing the same health problems we have.

I tell you this so, in your mind, you can begin placing healthy foods on one side of a scale and unhealthy foods on the other side. Look at the scale, point to the one with the wrong foods, and tell yourself it will age you. Then remind yourself that what is on the other side of the scale will make you healthy.

Granted, I would rather live in America than any other place I have ever visited or read about. But with a little knowledge, you can have the best of both worlds. You can have the same good health for your arteries as they do in such third world situations and at the same time enjoy all the privileges you have at home.

The Genetics Question

Genetics is overplayed in most minds. I have had patients tell me their Aunt Mary never exercised, ate butter, eggs, gravy, and fried potatoes all her life, and lived to be eighty-nine, so they can live a sedentary life because they have good genes. What they don't realize is that Aunt Mary may be the one in a thousand who survived that long but the studies show that the other 999 died before they should have. Plus, their last five years of life were terrible.

Don't even think about relying on good genes when contemplating a lifestyle of staying as young as possible. You are talking mountains and mole hills 99 percent of the time when you compare lifestyle and genetics. The other side of the coin, the bad genetic side, makes it even more important to develop your lifestyle properly. If you have a family history of heart disease, if one of your parents has had a heart attack at a young age (forty to sixty years old), there probably is a genetic factor at play. All that means is that you have to be even more committed to protect your arteries. So, either way, genetics is not a panacea for not working on your habits of health.

It Really Is about What You Eat

What you inherit is not nearly as significant as your present lifestyle. The medical literature includes many reports about people leaving a country where they were not eating foods high in saturated fat, trans fat, and dietary cholesterol and moving to America. Their cholesterol levels increase, resulting in a significant rise in the rate of heart attacks and strokes. A study showed Japanese men who moved from Japan to California or Hawaii ended up with a much higher cholesterol level, as well as a higher incidence of heart disease, than Japanese men living in Japan. The Japanese men who moved to the United States carried the same genes they always had, but their eating lifestyle changed to one that elevated their cholesterol level, which resulted in a higher incidence of heart disease. The more animal foods they ate, the higher their cholesterol became. They began eating steak and eggs. A lot of food had cheese added. Ice cream became routine. And a large percentage of what they ate was fried. It wasn't their genes that made the difference; it was in what they ate.

Medical statistics show that what you eat is the controlling factor of your physiological age. One report studied more than 1.5 million healthy adults who ate mainly whole-grain cereals, fruits, vegetables, nuts, pasta, fish, rice, and poultry. This group had a reduced risk of overall early mortality and cardiovascular mortality, as well as a reduced incidence of cancer and death from cancer. Here is the good part I liked: they also found a reduced incidence of Parkinson's and Alzheimer's disease.

Another study was performed on how many servings of fruits and vegetables you should eat. Is five a day better than one a day? Here is what was found in relation to stroke: *eating more than five servings of fruit a day reduced the risk of stroke by 25 percent*, as compared to those who ate fewer than three servings a day. Those figures make you want to place more fruit in your refrigerator for breakfast and snacks.

Let me close by encouraging you to continue changing your eating habits as we proceed. Set specific goals for yourself. You may not get your Total Cholesterol to 150 like reported in the African tribesmen, but your new eating strategy will prevent you from depositing splinters into your arteries. You will never have a heart attack or stroke or develop dementia caused by arterial disease. You may end up being killed by a lion, but when they perform your autopsy, they will find clean arteries. And if they use your heart as an example in a medical school anatomy class, yours will be the example of a strong heart with physiologically young arteries.

8

Grocery Shopping Made Easy

Someone once said they wished there was an app that allowed them to take a picture of the food they were thinking of buying at the grocery store that would then tell them whether or not they should eat it. Well, there is not an app like that (yet!), but there is something almost as easy. It is called the Nutrition Facts box. It tells you the serving size, calories, fat and sugar content, and sundry other facts. How do you pick the right foods at the grocery store? How do you know which ones you should never place in your cart? With these quick keys to the nutrition facts, you'll be ready to decide.

The initial step in defeating your eating addictions and habits is to not bring certain foods into your home. Winning the battle begins in the grocery store aisle. How you shop at the grocery store is one of the most important steps you can take to protect your arteries. It won't be long before you begin noticing that the foods in your cart are different from the ones you used to have in it. The day will come when you look at another person's cart and see all the cookies, hot dogs, and ice cream, and the absence of vegetables and fruits, and catch yourself wondering why they don't understand what they are doing to their bodies.

The Nutrition Facts box appears on every packaged food in America. It's on all of them: potato chips, crackers, packaged meats, canned soups, ice cream—everything. You don't have to look at all the numbers; just look at three of them. Once you have developed the habit of looking in the right spot for the right information, it will take less than ten seconds to decide whether to put the food in your cart or back on the shelf.

Nutrition Facts

Serving Size About 45 Crackers (30g)
Servings Per Container About 15

Amount Per Serving

Calories 120	Calories from Fat 0
	% Daily Value*
Total Fat 0g	**0%**
Saturated Fat 0g	**0%**
Trans Fat 0g	**0%**
Polyunsaturated Fat 0g	
Monounsaturated Fat 0g	
Cholesterol 0mg	**0%**
Sodium 400mg	**17%**
Total Carbohydrate 23g	**8%**
Dietary Fiber Less than 1g	**4%**
Sugars Less than 1g	
Protein 3g	
Vitamin A 0% • Vitamin C 0%	
Calcium 0% • Iron 8%	

*Percent Daily Values are based on a 2,000 calorie diet. Your daily values may be higher or lower depending on your calorie needs:

	Calories: 2,000	2,500
Total Fat	Less than 65g	80g
Sat Fat	Less than 20g	25g
Cholesterol	Less than 300mg	300mg
Sodium	Less than 2,400mg	2,400mg
Total Carbohydrate	300g	375g
Dietary Fiber	25g	30g

Calories per gram:
Fat 9 • Carbohydrate 4 • Protein 4

INGREDIENTS: ENRICHED WHEAT FLOUR (CONTAINS NIACIN, REDUCED IRON, THIAMINE MONONITRATE, RIBOFLAVIN AND FOLIC ACID), SALT, CORN SYRUP, MALT, YEAST, BICARBONATE AND CARBONATE OF SODIUM.

Whether you look at a box of club crackers or a bag of potato chips you will notice on the side of each container a label that shows in large print: Nutrition Facts.

This is what it looks like.

The diagram shows serving size, calories, different fats, sodium, total carbohydrates, dietary fiber, sugars, and protein.

Those are all interesting facts, but you can concentrate on one little section of the box. Train your eyes to go directly to the *total fat* and *cholesterol* segment of the box:

Nutrition Facts

Serving Size About 45 Crackers (30g)
Servings Per Container About 15

Amount Per Serving	
Calories 120	Calories from Fat 0
	% Daily Value*
Total Fat 0g	0%
Saturated Fat 0g	0%
Trans Fat 0g	0%
Polyunsaturated Fat 0g	
Monounsaturated Fat 0g	
Cholesterol 0mg	0%

You want to concentrate on the "bad threes." First, check the initial two items that are always listed directly under total fat: *saturated fat* and *trans fat*. In addition to those two, look for the dietary *cholesterol* number, which is always found just below the saturated fat and trans fat listing.

Zero, zero, zero is your target.

Saturated fat, trans fat, and dietary cholesterol are the most significant elements in foods that result in the greatest elevation of LDL Cholesterol in your blood. The rule is simple—look to see if there is any number other than zero beside each of these "bad threes," and if so, put the item back on the shelf and find a similar food that doesn't contain any of the "bad threes."

Train your eyes to look under total fat to find saturated fat and trans fat and just below that, cholesterol. Those "bad threes" are the ones to avoid like the plague.

For practice, let's go over some of the numbers you might see beside these items. If you examine two boxes of club crackers, one regular and one labeled "reduced fat," you will see something like this on the reduced fat box:

Nutrition Facts

Serving Size About 45 Crackers (30g)
Servings Per Container About 15

Amount Per Serving

Calories 120	Calories from Fat 0
	% Daily Value*
Total Fat 0g	0%
Saturated Fat 0g	0%
Trans Fat 0g	0%
Cholesterol 0mg	0%

Look under the Nutrition Facts section and see that saturated fat is zero, trans fat is zero, and cholesterol is zero. Zero, zero, zero; that's what you want. If you pick up the second box of club crackers, which looks identical to the first, except the "reduced fat" label is missing, you will see:

Nutrition Facts

Serving Size About 45 Crackers (30g)
Servings Per Container About 15

Amount Per Serving

Calories 120	Calories from Fat 0
	% Daily Value*
Total Fat 1.5g	0%
Saturated Fat 1.5g	0%
Trans Fat 0g	0%
Cholesterol 0mg	0%

This box of crackers reads saturated fat 1.5g, trans fat 0g, and cholesterol 0mg. It takes less than ten seconds to remember that the one fat we as Americans eat the most of, the one that raises our LDL Cholesterol, is *saturated fat*. It's found in so many of our foods that you can't believe it.

If you develop that simple ten-second shopping step of knowing where to look on the Nutrition Facts box, you are off to the races. You *will* find food choices that are similar to what you want but have lower saturated fat content; all you need to do is look. Plus, the good part is, if you were to take crackers out of both boxes and mix them, it would be difficult to tell a difference in taste—especially if you are eating the cracker with a bowl of soup or with something on the cracker. If you weren't watching for the saturated fat, trans fat, and cholesterol content, you could pick up the nonreduced fat crackers without thinking anything about it and eat the lethal enemy. And if you multiply that one example by all the items you buy without observing the "bad threes," you will end up bringing into your home a whole bag full of enemies. It doesn't seem all that significant, but it is.

I don't want to make it sound too simple, because you will find many, many foods with zero trans fat and zero cholesterol, but the saturated fat section is where you will have the most difficult time finding a zero. You will not find triple zeros on many items, but it will surprise you how often you will find them—if you look. Let's look more at each of the "bad threes."

Trans fat. In reality, you will find a zero beside the trans fat almost every time. Trans fat is so bad that the government has recently moved to ban it. However, occasionally, you will find some trans fat listed, and the rule for trans fat is absolute zero. Trans fat? Put it back. Do not falter from that one. Remember that trans fat is the one used as a preservative and is (or was) found in those foods at the corner market where the goods sit on a shelf for a long period of time—cookies, donuts, pastries, and the like.

Cholesterol. Most food manufacturers have come to realize the danger of using cholesterol in their baking or cooking process, and the majority of times, cholesterol will also be zero. However, it is still not unusual to find cholesterol listed in cookies, candies, and pastries and such. Although dietary cholesterol is not as lethal as trans fat, you still need to make cholesterol an absolute zero. If there is a number other than zero beside cholesterol, put the item back. Ninety-nine percent of the time, if you look, you will be able to find a similar food with trans fat and cholesterol being zero.

Saturated fat. Now we come to the reality of saturated fat. A zero is what you aim for, but you will not be able to find everything you want within that limit. You may have to bump your desired number from zero up to 0.5 grams. The goal is still zero, but reality makes us allow a 0.5 gram number. Most candy bars and similar foods will range from 2 to 7 grams—so they are out. Develop a different desire for such foods. Aim for a saturated fat of zero, but for practicality, a half a gram is permissible. Develop your habit. If over 0.5 grams for saturated fat, put the item back. And that's not 5; it's 0.5.

Take a minute to learn these numbers because you want to develop the habit of looking for them each time you pick up a packaged item of food, whether at the grocery store or in the fast-food market. Let's say you want potato chips or something similar to go with a sandwich. You look in the grocery store and find a bag that says "reduced fat." Look at the Nutrition Facts box and see zero, zero, zero for saturated fat, trans fat, and cholesterol.

However, your children or grandchildren want those reddish-coated Doritos chips so they can get that red on their fingers and lick it off. You look at regular Doritos and see saturated fat: 1.5g with zero trans fat and zero cholesterol. Next to that group of bags you see another group of bags of Doritos that look the same on the picture, but on the bag it says "baked." Looking at the Nutrition Facts box, you find zero beside the trans fat and cholesterol, and under saturated fat you see 0.5g. The regular Doritos have three times the amount of saturated fat as the baked ones. You simply pick up the baked product and let your grandchildren begin developing the habit of eating their favorite chips—baked. That's what I'm talking about. Begin looking at the Nutrition Facts box and choose the foods you actually want to take home.

You will see figures that are completely out of reach in some foods you routinely had in your kitchen pantry at one time, such as packaged foods like donuts and cakes, with saturated fat at 9 to 12 grams, perhaps a couple of grams of trans fat, and a lot of cholesterol. Those are the foods you won't touch with a ten-foot pole anymore, much less take them home with you.

In the weight-loss part of the plan, you won't be eating snacks between meals. But once you reach your ideal weight, the snack basics you will buy at the store will consist of nuts and fruits. That's it. So start your new habits by buying some nuts and bananas, grapes, oranges, blueberries, cherries, strawberries, or any other fruit you like. After you're at your ideal weight and want a snack, reach for a fruit, some nuts, or a combination of the two. Nuts contain saturated fat, but they contain a great deal more of the good fats than the bad (and that's good).

9

Foods to Avoid

A friend of mine told me about a drastic change his brother made in the overall lifestyle he was living. "He smoked and drank too much. He was forty years old, overweight, and had elevated blood pressure." It was almost as though he was bragging about all the bad his brother did. "His doctor, rather forcefully, informed him that if he didn't give up drinking and smoking and get to a normal weight, he would be dead in five years. From that *moment* on, he never took one sip of alcohol, never took one draw on a cigarette, and he lost all his excess weight. And now, twenty years later, he is still vibrant."

Cigarettes and alcohol might not be a problem for you. But everyone has to eat. And everyone should eat the right foods if they want to live younger longer.

I want to create a mind picture you should never forget, one that will help you remember what foods to avoid. I won't go so far as to say it is a picture of foods you will *never* eat again; I won't ask you to become fanatical about it. But you need a clear understanding of what these foods do to your arteries. You will learn how to change your desire for these foods into a desire for more healthy foods. You will learn which foods keep your body, heart, and mind young.

Let me say again that I care how long you live, but I care even more about how young you keep your body and mind until that day eventually comes. You will indeed add years to your life on this plan, but that is secondary. More important, you will learn how to add life to your years. You want to be as active as possible up until that very last day.

Here is your picture of foods *not* to eat.

A Big, Juicy Steak

Picture yourself sitting at a nice restaurant as the waiter brings an oval platter and sets it directly in front of you. On it he places a big, juicy steak. This image stands for red meat: beef, in addition to the pork and lamb you are going to avoid. The saturated fat is highest in these meats, and you are going to begin avoiding them when choosing what you eat. In fact, the day will come when you won't even want to buy or order them because your *desires* will change.

You hear that center-cut bacon, which is cut next to the bone, has less saturated fat than other bacon. You hear of leaner cuts of beef having less fat than others. You even hear how grass-fed beef is much better for you than all others. All that may well be true to a minute degree, but what you want to imprint in your mind is that certain foods are dangerous to your arteries and other foods are not. I won't argue the point of one being a little lower in saturated fat than another, because we are not discussing minutia. You are learning changes in your eating lifestyle. You are learning a habit of avoiding certain food types. You want to begin avoiding the types of foods that contain the saturated fat that is known to rob you of your health.

The steak picture is associated with red meat, but you must also remind yourself of bacon. Bacon is the one meat in which you can actually see the layers of fat. Focus on the fat in bacon whenever you see a strip cooking or someone eating it. If you are eating bacon, you are eating fat. There is over a gram of fat per strip of bacon. You talk about addiction—someone who loved bacon told me he used to think bacon was bad for him, so he just gave up thinking.

Eating red meat increases your overall risk of disease in the arteries of your heart as well as causes an increased risk of certain cancers. There is a double-blind study of more than half a million people. In one group, individuals ate red meat and processed meat, and in the other group, individuals limited their intake of meat to white meat. The researchers compared death from cancer as well as disease to the arteries of their hearts and found an overall increased risk of cancer and coronary vascular disease in those who ate the greatest amount of red meat.

Here is the bottom line: the study showed the health risks of diets loaded with red meat, such as hamburger and steak, and processed meats, such as hot dogs, bacon, and cold cuts. They found that over a ten-year period, men who ate the equivalent of a quarter-pounder hamburger a day had a 22 percent higher risk of dying from cancer and a 27 percent higher risk of dying from heart disease than those men whose diet did not contain such red meat.

With women, it was even more impressive. Women who ate large amounts of red meat had a 20 percent higher risk of dying from cancer and a 50 percent higher risk of dying from heart disease.

Think of these numbers every time you are tempted to stray from the Prescription for Life plan.

And remember, this was a study of more than five hundred thousand people. It's not complicated. One group ate red meat and the other didn't. Such studies should make a lasting impression on you every time you are offered a hot dog at a ball game or asked by wait staff if you want sausage to go with your egg-white veggie omelet. Imagine putting a steak on one side of the scale and a piece of salmon on the other side and asking yourself which side gives you a much greater risk of heart disease and cancer and which side is protecting your health. Which side of the scale are you going to eat from?

This same report from the *Archives of Internal Medicine* goes into even more interesting detail. Some within that group who ate the greatest amount of red meat changed their eating lifestyle and began eating the same as the group who ate very little red meat. *The study found that there was an 11 percent decrease in early mortality in the men and a 21 percent decrease in early mortality in the women who changed to the healthy diet.*

What a dramatic finding about the effect red meat has on our arteries. This shows that even if you are a heavy-red-meat-eating person, you can decrease your early mortality rate by decreasing the amount of red meat you eat. It shows you can change your eating lifestyle now and protect your arteries for years to come.

One other article gives a great example about finding a healthy substitute food to replace a damaging food. This study followed more than one hundred thousand people for more than twenty years. The study was about death rate—mortality—and showed that the amount of red meat eaten was linked to an increase in risk for premature death. The more red meat eaten, the earlier the death toll. The researchers even took it further and compared the individuals who ate fish or chicken with the ones who ate red meat. In every situation, it was found to be advantageous to eat something other than red meat.

Here is the encouraging part of the study—it links what you're learning about your cholesterol numbers with a significant finding. This study showed that Total Cholesterol and Low Density Lipoprotein Cholesterol levels were decreased in people who substituted fish for red meat.

I will eat red meat several times a year. When I go to Alaska for a week or two in March, the people I eat with cook a lot of steak on the grill. They usually grill a chicken breast for me, but when that runs out, I will eat a steak—or at least half of one. If I am at a banquet or a home where only steak is served, I will eat some. You don't have to be fanatical to develop a proper lifestyle of eating. My basic eating strategy is to not eat red meat. And that wasn't my lifestyle growing up. In college and med school and for many years later, I ate red meat numerous times a week. That was my habit of eating.

I heard about the difference between being ignorant and stupid and applied it to eating red meat. Before I read the medical literature about red meat, I was ignorant of the harm it did as I ate it. But after hearing the statistics, I don't want to consider myself stupid by continuing to eat it.

Fried Egg Sunny Side Up: On Top of the Steak

Your waiter comes by and adds a fried egg, sunny side up, on top of the steak on the platter. Egg yolk is one of the highest cholesterol foods there is, with one jumbo egg yolk containing 270mg of dietary cholesterol. Egg yolks contribute about one-third of the dietary cholesterol in the food supply of what we eat. Compare that to four ounces of beef, containing 100mg, and salmon with only 70mg, and better than that, to four ounces of tuna with only 40mg. Looking at these examples, you see it is pretty simple to choose tuna or salmon over steak and eggs for any meal. Don't overlook a simple egg when you are talking dietary cholesterol. It is used so much in cooking. It is almost impossible to eat in America and not eat egg yolks, especially if you eat baked goods.

Your three main sources of dietary cholesterol in America are eggs, red meat, and cheese. The bottom line still reminds you that the intake of dietary cholesterol raises the LDL in your blood.

Don't confuse "dietary cholesterol" with the "cholesterol" mentioned in your lab cholesterol numbers. Dietary cholesterol is one of the three food sources that can raise your LDL Cholesterol within your body, with saturated fat and trans fat being the other two. Each of these food types alone raises the LDL Cholesterol in your blood. But most of the bad foods you eat have a mixture of these "bad threes." I said egg yolks have more cholesterol than steak—but I also remind you that steak has more saturated fat than egg yolks. Don't try to separate each bad factor out by itself. Learn which foods to avoid whether they contain cholesterol alone, saturated fat alone, or a mixture.

You can cook or order an egg-white veggie omelet—no yolk. You won't get the dietary cholesterol if you leave out the yolk. But remember, when you order the egg-white omelet, specify that you don't want any cheese. I tell you this because, about half the time, they will automatically add cheese unless you specify no cheese, and you may end up with an omelet loaded with saturated fat cheese. As my grandfather told me, if something has a fifty-fifty chance of going wrong, nine times out of ten it will. If you order toast to go with the omelet, tell them you want plain, dry toast. If you don't, there's a fifty-fifty chance they will bring it to you drenched in butter. And by the way, you won't be eating the ham or bacon or sausage that usually comes with a breakfast, even if they do bring it to the table.

How do you cook without egg yolks? One cook told me to use just one more egg than called for and to use only the whites. Another said you could substitute applesauce for eggs. Another very confidently stated she used egg substitutes like eggbeaters. She states that on the package of egg substitutes it tells you exactly how much to use for each egg substituted. She stated no one could tell the difference between the real and the substitute. I give you these hints from people who cook, but I can't tell you authoritatively because I am not a cook. I manage to burn toast in a toaster, for some reason.

I introduce this next "food to avoid" by asking you a question. Do you know what one food consumed in America contains the greatest amount of animal fat? I have gotten many answers to this question, including steak, sausage, pork, ice cream, and desserts. But they are all wrong. I have mentioned it before, but in case you don't recall, the answer is cheese. There is more animal fat eaten in cheese than in any other food. Lethal Low Density Lipoprotein—LDL—is what you are elevating in your bloodstream when you eat cheese.

Cheese: On Top of the Steak and Egg

The waiter places a big slice of cheese squarely on top of the steak and the sunny-side-up egg. Watch as the yolk breaks—the yellow runs out between the cheese and the steak and flows down onto the platter. As a matter of fact, there is such a large yolk puddle on the platter that it appears the steak is floating in yellow yolk.

As I told you in an earlier chapter, at one time, cheese was one of my most favorite foods. My patients knew how much I liked it and brought me all types of cheese as Christmas gifts. Then I read a journal article explaining that cheese is the most eaten food in America that has the most saturated fat of any food. The article went on to point out how the saturated fat in cheese causes an increase in LDL Cholesterol, which is a primary cause of blockage in arteries of the heart. By the time I finished reading the medical journal article, I had made the decision to quit eating cheese. *I hope you have just made the same decision.*

Whole Milk: Glass to Right of Platter

In your mind, picture the steak on the platter, a soft-cooked egg on top of the steak, with a slice of cheese lying on the egg. Now see your waiter place a glass of whole milk beside the right upper portion of the platter. If you look closely, you will see little specks of pure cream floating on top of the milk. Milk and cream: both dairy products. Milk is rich in nutrients and the calcium your bones need. The bad part: milk contains a great deal of fat. The good part: we can easily buy, drink, and cook using milk that has the fat removed.

Whole milk contains about 4 percent butterfat. That reads as 6 grams of saturated fat on the Nutrition Facts label. Skim milk has all the fat removed. It doesn't take a genius to figure it out. If you want to decrease the amount of fat you put into your body, begin using skim milk—or almond milk or soy milk—on a routine basis.

Look at it this way: you and your family are going to drink whatever is in the refrigerator. That could be whole milk or skim milk. Your family drinks whatever is bought at the grocery store. You don't have to change their drinking habits; you just have to change your buying habits.

I recall when I first realized how much fat was in milk. It was stunning to me, as a physician. I read that the fat I would consume while drinking a glass of whole milk is equivalent to eating five strips of bacon. I couldn't even imagine how much fat was in a half gallon of whole milk. I don't know why certain little statements like that made me change my eating lifestyle, but the more I thought about it, the more I began to reason that I should cut back on whole milk consumption. I will never forget drinking my first glass of skim milk. It felt and tasted like water. I was sure it was a taste I would never grow to like. But I kept thinking about fatty bacon, and it wasn't too long before skim milk tasted "normal" and a sip of whole milk made me wonder why I ever liked it in the first place.

If you look at a quart of whole milk that has not been pasteurized, you will see that the cream has risen to the top of the container. Whole milk you buy in the store contains that same amount of pure cream, just mixed in with the rest of the milk. So when you think of milk, you have to also include that cream in your mind picture.

That takes ice cream out of your eating lifestyle.

As well as cream sauces restaurants want to pour over your grilled fish.

As well as cream-based soups you eat because you forgot to ask if the soup you were ordering was cream based or not.

As well as so many desserts that taste so good.

I know you may be thinking right now, "No way." But I have told you about my father and the blockage of his coronary artery and the blockage of his intestinal artery that was his fatal blow. He ate mostly healthy, including vegetables and fruits. Very, very seldom did I ever see him eat a steak. But one thing my mother would get for him every night was a bowl of ice cream. He loved ice cream. That is the only food I can think of that he ate on a regular basis that was full of those little LDL Cholesterol splinters.

If cheese was the most difficult food for me to give up when I realized I needed to change my eating lifestyle, ice cream was the second most difficult.

So with the glass of milk to the upper right side of your platter, you have to remind yourself it contains more than just the milk. You emphasize the cream within the milk and think ice cream, cream cheese, whipped cream, cream sauces, cream-based soup, and anything else in which cream is used.

Butter: Patty to the Left of the Plate

The waiter now places a pat of butter on a small plate on the upper left side of the platter. Butter has two of the sources of the bad kind of food you want to avoid. It has both dietary cholesterol as well as dietary saturated fat.

Many say to substitute margarine for butter because margarine doesn't contain dietary cholesterol. And they are half right but still half wrong. Although margarine doesn't have the dietary cholesterol butter contains, it still has about the same amount of saturated fat as butter. Butter and margarine both fit into the "bad" picture. So quit putting either butter or margarine on your bread and your baked potato.

Rather than butter or margarine, use substitutes like Benecol or Promise activ. These are cholesterol-lowering spreads. Also, use olive oil and canola oil in cooking. They contain the good monounsaturated and polyunsaturated fats. If you want to put something on your bread, put some olive oil on it.

Many of the sauces put on the foods you order are butter or cream based. A simple question to ask yourself is whether or not the sauce is cream based. You may order grilled fish for your dinner, but with it comes a thick cream-based sauce that is butter loaded. You will learn to avoid the creamy Alfredo sauce and ask for a marinara or basil sauce instead. Once you learn who the enemy is, you will think completely differently about what foods you eat.

Fried

For the final piece in our picture, your waiter brings out a small plate with a polished silver bowl in the center and sets it before you on the table. You look into it and see a blob of grease. He then picks up the bowl and pours it, first on the butter, then into the glass of milk, and then the rest onto the top of the slice of cheese. Part of it splatters onto the tablecloth while the rest runs down over the egg and steak and mixes with the yellow egg yolk floating on the bottom of the platter. He places the little silver bowl back on the platter and walks away.

As he leaves, he turns his head and states two words: "Nothing fried."

What a great reminder. The basic oil mostly used today in frying food is animal based and full of the saturated fat you want to avoid. That silver bowl of grease represents a lot of foods you now eat. But from this day on, you want to put these fried foods on a scale and weigh the outcome of what will happen to the arteries in your heart and brain if you continue consuming them as you now do. Just think of all the fried foods you eat. French fries, fried fish, fried chicken, and the list goes on and on. Down South, they even eat fried green tomatoes. To learn from this portion of the picture, begin thinking *grilled* rather than fried. Whether cooking at home or placing your order at a restaurant, begin developing your strategy of choosing grilled rather than fried foods. It will become an easy rule to follow. When you see the word *fried* on a menu, you look further.

But just because you order grilled doesn't mean you have protected your arteries. You also have to be aware of the type of sauces they are going to place on top of your grilled fish or chicken, or on any other entrée. You ask the type of sauce used because you do not want one that is cream or cheese based. A simple way to order is to ask that all sauces be placed on the side. Then you can determine whether it is a cheese sauce or cream or butter based, and if so, you leave it sitting beside your plate.

If you are cooking foods at home, use oils that are high in the good fat. The "good three" fats are the ones high in mono-unsaturated and polyunsaturated fats. They are found in the canola oils and olive oils. Some restaurants use such oils in frying foods, but the majority use the oils that are high in saturated fat. Think grilled rather than fried, not only because of the bad oils used in the frying but also because frying a food adds about a third more calories than grilling the same food. Grilling cuts down on calories as well as saturated fat.

The waiter is gone, and now you have the picture. It will help you remember about 90 percent of the foods you are going to eliminate from your eating lifestyle. This makes it easier to follow through in making your eating habit changes. (Even if you try to forget the picture, for some reason, you will always remember it.) You don't have to quit them all at once, but you want to begin working on the entire picture.

A gentleman was interested in learning what foods he should be avoiding to protect his health and asked me for some advice.

I didn't go through the entire Prescription for Life plan but only explained the "save your life" picture you just learned. I saw him in a group of people two days later, and he waved me over.

"Last night I got to thinking about what you explained concerning the danger of saturated fat, trans fat, and dietary cholesterol," he said. "I just want you to know what I did. I took a gallon container of Blue Bell ice cream out of my freezer and threw it in the trash. It was my favorite ice cream; 28 percent butterfat type. But I threw it away." He laughed and walked on back to the group he was with.

He looked back at me. "Just wanted you to know."

Here's another story about avoiding the wrong foods.

A gentleman took my wife and me to dinner the other night. His father had a heart attack at age fifty-eight. His wife sat quietly as he told us his own experience of chest pain one evening that ended with him in the ER. He went downhill quickly, and he needed to be air lifted to a larger medical center nearby. But fog had moved into the mountainous area, and he had to ride an hour and a half down the mountain by ambulance. The blocked artery was not accessible for a stent to be placed, and he underwent emergency coronary artery bypass.

The operation was a success, but six months later, he was sitting at the table telling me what his cholesterol numbers are. His HDL is fairly low, and even on medication, his LDL is still high. We went to our home after dinner, and I took his blood pressure. It was dangerously elevated. He was on blood pressure medication, but his doctor cut it in half two months ago to see if his pressure could remain down with less medication. He was not what you would consider obese, but he was about twenty-five pounds overweight. The conversation that followed was not a pretty one as I explained what he must do to prevent passing on early, leaving his wife and children without the guidance of a husband and a father. He immediately stated he would do anything to prolong his life. He said: "Anything—eating—not eating—weight control—whatever. Just tell me."

I asked his wife what his favorite foods were, and she replied, "Steak and cheese." I immediately turned to him and said, "You have just eaten your last piece of cheese." I have never seen a more earnest-looking face as he nodded repeatedly.

"Anything you say," was his quick reply. His next question was, "What else?" I knew he had just realized what he was up against and was willing to pay whatever it took to be able to live longer and healthier. I went over the food picture I just shared with you. I went over the breakdown of cholesterol. I explained the LDL Cholesterol splinters and where they came from. I went over the significance of normal weight in relation to his blood pressure and LDL cholesterol. I went over an exercise program for him. All this, in about fifteen minutes. I have never in my life seen an individual with such a fear of the results of a wrong lifestyle. He seized the moment. Following the discussion, his first statement to his wife was, "No more cheese."

Like me, no more cheese was his initial step. It only takes a moment to decide you are going to commit. I know, because it only took one single medical article about the damage cheese causes to my arteries for me to commit to quit eating my favorite food.

All this happened after his doctor gave him the ultimatum concerning what was aging him. It took only a *moment* for him to decide and commit to change his lifestyle—forever.

This is what I want the Prescription for Life plan to do. The vast majority who sign on to commit to changing their lifestyle will do so once they realize how to do it—and why. It is so exciting to see individuals make the commitment to change a part of their lifestyle, especially when it involves throwing away a favorite ice cream they have eaten almost nightly for years.

Now, with a picture fixed in your mind of what you will choose *not* to eat, let's look at the specific foods you *will* choose to eat—for the rest of your life.

10

Foods to Live By

You hear about so many diets, and it is difficult to know which is best. Many of them are medically sound for the particular problem you may have, so if your physician has placed you on a special diet, by all means, follow your doctor's advice.

But your Prescription for Life plan is about you and the rest of your life.

You want an eating plan that has staying power. Some plans cut down on sugar. Some deal with the glycemic index. And the list for specific targets to avoid goes on and on. Then there are the ones that will cause you to lose weight but are detrimental to your health. One in particular has you eating protein only—but it is full of the saturated fat and cholesterol that plug your arteries. Such types may get weight off but play havoc with your arteries. Then there are the ones that are indeed healthy but are not what you are going to be able to continue following for the rest of your life.

Some people drink a homemade smoothie that is filled with all kinds of good fruits and even some vegetables, but the problem is that such a diet is usually not something you can maintain when you travel, and it may not be something you can maintain for the rest of your life. I questioned a friend concerning this, and he said he planned on drinking a smoothie for breakfast from now on. (I didn't argue. It will be great if he actually does.)

Others eat certain kinds of bars for breakfast. And even others buy into a preplanned diet program in which the food is delivered through the mail. I have seen such a diet plan work wonders in getting the weight off, but again the question remains, Is it a lifestyle you can sustain for the rest of your life? The lifestyle you can sustain begins at the grocery store, but now we move to the step beyond grocery shopping. This is where the rubber meets the road—the basic foods to eat, and not to eat, whether you are eating at home or in a restaurant.

A healthy diet protects your arteries. Recently published in the *Annals of Neurology*, a study conducted exams on seven hundred people who were sixty-five or older. Those who adhered more closely to a diet consisting mainly of fruits and vegetables, whole-grain bread, pasta, olive oil, and fish were up to 36 percent less likely to have damage to their brains as a result of small strokes.

That's good news for those following the Prescription for Life plan.

Prescription for Life Foods

Let's begin with the types of foods you'll enjoy with the Prescription for Life plan. The diet platform begins with an emphasis on vegetables and fruits. You are encouraged to aim for a combination of five fruits and vegetables per day. You get most of the fruits with your breakfast, as well as fruits and nuts for snack time.

In addition to fruits and vegetables, you are also encouraged to think whole grains. Think of whole-grain cereal in the morning, whole-grain breads for sandwiches, whole-grain pasta for an evening meal, or rice with sautéed vegetables or fish chunks on top.

Choose olive oil or canola oil for cooking. Get away from oils derived from animal fat, because they are high in saturated fat or trans fat that is partially hydrogenated. Even though olive oil is a fat and does contain nine calories per gram, it contains a lot of monounsaturated fat. This is one of your good three fat that help limit LDL Cholesterol and also raise your HDL Cholesterol.

If you have a desire for meat, go with fish first and then grilled chicken. Those two will take the place of red meat from now on. You won't go to the extreme, learning a list of fish in descending order according to the amount of omega-3 fatty acid each has. But you will change your eating lifestyle of hamburgers, steak, and barbecue pork to eating more fish. Now, that's not extreme, is it?

So major on fruits, vegetables, and salads with peas, legumes, and beans.

Beware of the diets that say you can still eat some "bad" if you do so in moderation. The Prescription for Life plan encourages you to run from the "bad" so you won't continue having the desire for such foods. So many diets encourage you to eat foods containing saturated fat, trans fat, and dietary cholesterol in "moderation." They encourage you to eat cheese in moderation or to use low-fat cheese. This sets you up to continue having the desire for such foods.

Healthy Choices for Every Meal

What kinds of foods should you choose for each meal in your new, healthy lifestyle? The following suggestions are only a few examples of what you can eat. I'll explain why a particular food is a good foundation for your eating habits, but you may try other foods as long as you stick to the principles you have been learning.

When you finish this section, you will have good ideas of what to eat for each meal. I want you to build a platform meal for breakfast, lunch, and dinner. Each platform will consist of a list of basic foods you will use as a foundation for that particular meal. You should develop the habit of eating your three platform meals every day for a three-week period. Keep it simple. Then you can add a second or third alternate tier to your initial platform. Again, these alternate tiers will follow the same rules you made for your basic platform diet, but they will allow you to have additional selections of what to eat. But as you begin, I would like for you to choose from the foods listed here to build your basic platform diet for each meal of the day.

All three platform meals avoid saturated fat, trans fat, and dietary cholesterol—and emphasize high fiber cereals, fruit, whole grains, vegetables, salads, peas, legumes, beans, nuts, pasta, fish, and chicken.

The most important aspect of the Prescription for Life strategy for eating is that your platform diet will be the same whether you are considering losing weight or maintaining your ideal weight. You will change to smaller portions when you are losing weight, and you may eat some between meal snacks after you are at your ideal weight, but the basic rules of what foods you will eat and what foods you will avoid remain the same.

Your platform diet will consist of the basic foods that will automatically come to mind when you think of a particular meal. Your platform diet will become the basis of what you will end up desiring to eat. Your platform diet will be foods you will form an addiction to. And that will be a good addiction.

First of all, you will eat three meals a day. Even if you are going to be losing weight, the three meals a day rule is in order. Studies show that nearly 80 percent of people who lose weight and keep it off eat breakfast every day. You will be eating three meals a day after you have reached your ideal weight goal, so you need to form the lifestyle of eating three meals a day as you lose weight to get there.

A friend of mine had been gaining weight slowly, but year after year of gain resulted in him being obese. I would see him every so often, sometimes not for six or eight months. But one day we both attended the same meeting, and I was shocked to see he had gained at least another twenty pounds since I had last seen him. At the meeting, I happened to be following him as we approached a flight of stairs. I watched as he went up. It was more of a waddle than stair climbing. His legs were so big that his knees barely flexed. He nearly pulled the handrail off its wall braces. He had started wearing his shirttail pulled out in an attempt to hide his stomach, but even then his protruding abdomen pushed a nice roundness right through the front. I could not believe he had gained so much weight since the last time I saw him. He told me his doctor was referring him to an orthopedist for knee replacements. He didn't look happy.

I made a decision. That evening, I sat him down and told him that he was going to do one of two things. "Either you are going to change your lifestyle, which will include eating habits, exercise, and losing weight, or I am going to set you up for a gastric bypass operation—which won't work unless you change your whole mentality about your physical condition." I didn't want to sound harsh, but the time had come for him to face reality—something had to be done. "You are killing yourself, and if you don't do something about it, you will not be able to walk within this coming year." I was adamant with my friend of many years. I told him to talk it over with his wife and decide between surgery and lifestyle change, assuring him that I was not going to stand by and let a good friend go downhill like he was.

The next morning at breakfast, he and his wife said the decision had been made to change his eating lifestyle. I am going to use my friend's lifestyle diet to teach you the basic platform diet you can develop. Here is where we started, and you can begin making specific goals for your own eating lifestyle. Less than a year later, he has lost sixty pounds, is jogging and lifting weights on a regular basis, and can walk up a flight of stairs as quickly as I can.

Breakfast: The Easiest Platform

The rule of thumb for breakfast is to aim for a combination of five fruits and vegetables a day or a total of five fruits a day. Breakfast is the easiest time to get in over half your fruits. A high fiber cereal—and equally important, fruit—will become your mainstay for breakfast. Add any three fruits to your cereal—bananas, strawberries, and blueberries go well together. For your remaining fruits for the rest of the day, keep apples and oranges on your counter and grapes in your refrigerator, plus any other favorites you may have.

Breakfast is the easiest meal to set into your new lifestyle of eating. Fiber is one of the best foods you can eat for a good intestinal tract. Not only does fiber help protect you against colon cancer, but it also improves bowel movements. A high fiber breakfast will give you a regularity that will take care of any constipation you may have. It regulates your bowels because fiber is not easily absorbed. It moves through your intestines quicker and, at the same time, absorbs water in your colon, making your stools soft. Without the straining associated with constipation, there is less buildup of pressure within the colon that commonly results in small out-pouching of the wall of the colon. These little out-pouches are about as large as the end of your little finger and are called diverticula. These can become infected and cause what is termed diverticulitis, or they can rupture and require an operation.

The *British Medical Journal* reported that those who eat more than 25 grams of fiber a day have a 41 percent reduced risk of being hospitalized or dying of diverticulitis complications when compared to individuals who ate less than 14 grams of fiber daily. The medical literature emphasizes that eating fiber is the best protection against diverticulosis or diverticulitis. You don't have to remember the numbers; just remember that fiber is a big protector of your colon in many ways. (We will discuss how it protects against colon cancer later.) Make a commitment to eat more fiber.

You will get most of your fiber from your breakfast, but it is also good to remember it throughout the day. You hear a lot about whole grain being good for you. The reason is because of the amount of fiber in whole grain. Most of the fiber in grain comes from the outer covering, the kernel. Refining the grain strips away the fiber.

Cereal alternatives include steel-cut oats as your oatmeal. The difference between regular oatmeal and steel-cut is that steel-cut has the outer covering left intact. Choose whole-grain breads at the grocery store. Choose brown rice, which still has the kernel on it, instead of white rice. You can even find whole-grain pasta.

There are several ways to increase your fiber throughout the day, but breakfast is still the simplest and easiest meal in which to get the most total fiber at one time.

So many patients come back to me throughout the years and thank me for advising them on such a simple high fiber breakfast plan for their bowel habits. They are so thankful that they have a single soft, simple, normal bowel movement each morning without any problem. You may get a chuckle from that—but of all the suggestions I have made to patients, this is the one that patients have told me time and again they appreciate. They are so thankful I talked to them about regulating their bowels.

I will suggest several cereals as examples for what you can choose. Not everyone will be able to eat the most high fiber content cereals, but I encourage you to eat the highest fiber content you can. Next time you choose a cereal from the grocery store, look at the Nutrition Facts section on the box and see how much fiber that particular cereal contains. I will give you some examples: Cheerios shows 3 grams, while Honey Bunches of Oats shows 2 grams, and Raisin Bran goes up to 7 grams. Now, I want to tell you my favorite—the one that contains the highest fiber content of all our common cereals. And that is whole-grain Fiber One. It comes in different types, and the fiber content ranges from 13 to 17 grams per serving. Going by fiber content, eating one bowl of Fiber One is similar to eating five bowls of Cheerios. That is a good lifestyle breakfast to begin your day—using skim milk, of course. And add on a lot of strawberries and/or bananas and/or blueberries and/or raspberries, or any other fruit you may like on cereals.

So your primary platform breakfast will be a high fiber cereal like Fiber One, with lots of fruits and skim milk.

As a side note, almond milk is zero, zero, zero nondairy. No saturated fat, no trans fat, and no dietary cholesterol. You can also use soy milk, rice milk—any of those without the butterfat. I recommend skim milk because everyone knows about it and even husbands can find it in the grocery store.

If you are tired of cereal one morning and want to cook or order a different breakfast, go for an egg-white veggie omelet with whole-grain toast and jelly of some sort. Some say egg-beaters are quicker to fix.

If you want more alternatives, you can make them up yourself with such ideas as nonfat yogurt with fruit. Or some people have made a habit of making a smoothie using frozen fruits. They keep a stash of the fruit in their freezer, and a smoothie is their daily breakfast. They can even drink it on the way to work. I will admit that I tried frozen smoothies once, but they just didn't have the taste I thought they ought to. So I just kept eating my Fiber One cereal. However, I do have several friends who say that is what they like, and they plan to drink one every morning for years to come.

Oatmeal is another food you can add to your breakfast secondary platform. You can add raisins, cinnamon, yogurt, or strawberries or blueberries. You can eat it dry or add skim milk. There are all sorts of combinations you can develop as an alternative to high fiber cereal. And remember that steel-cut has more fiber.

And there is that old quick, in a hurry, got to get to the office toast and jelly. Whole-grain toast, and dry—that is, without adding butter. You just put some of your favorite jelly on it, eat it, and go.

Concerning what to drink with all this, most people have coffee. Breakfast is also a good time for high pulp orange juice. The juice is not as good for you as the whole fruit, but it is still good. The high pulp has the most fiber. If you are in the weight-loss stage of your diet, you may want to skip the orange juice because it gives you extra calories.

Remember, breakfast is easy—fiber and fruit. You can easily get three of your five daily fruits at breakfast time.

Lunch: Keep It Simple

Now that you know vegetables and fruits are your mainstays, if I were to ask you to choose your own primary lunch platform, I hope you would think of salad. You probably don't believe it, but you can build a lot on a salad as your primary base platform for lunch—as long as you don't add any cheese and always use a fat-free dressing.

Vegetables give you the most food content with the fewest calories. They give you a feeling of being satisfactorily full. You can eat an unlimited amount of vegetables. Weight Watchers has been successful over the years by having you count points for the foods you eat. Recently, they came out with a new rule that you can eat all the vegetables you want—completely point free except for a few, like peas and corn, and those are still very low in points. The reason for this is because such foods satisfy your hunger with the fewest calories. Your stomach will be stuffed, and it will be with food that gives you the most nourishment with the fewest calories possible. What more can you want than to feel full and not have paid the calorie price to do so?

There are numerous salad lunches you can eat, especially if you are eating out. Even fast-food restaurants have an assortment of salads now, including with strawberries and fat-free dressings. As you get into it, you will find more and more ways of eating a salad at lunch. I remind you to guard against letting them put cheese on the salad, and you must also remember to use a fat-free dressing. Always ask for the dressing to be placed on the side rather than on the salad. That way you control the amount you use. It is a shame to sit at a restaurant and watch someone put cups of salad

Eat the Right Foods

dressing on their salad and then sprinkle cheese all over it. High fat dressings can add up to four hundred calories, and sprinkled cheese can add another hundred. Even more significant than the additional calories is the saturated fat being added.

If you are in the weight-loss stage of lifestyle eating, salad is definitely your base platform. I say that because you will want to eat a double or triple salad rather than begin adding foods that have greater calories per gram than the vegetables in the salad.

Once you have reached your ideal weight, you can choose foods to add to your basic lunch platform. A simple addition is grilled fish or grilled chicken. You will be adding them in small portions to your salad rather than as a full entrée, but you will be getting different tastes to your salads from time to time.

Also, in the same way, you can add a nondairy-based soup to the meal. No cream-based soup is ever allowed, but a bowl of soup can add a nice variety to your meal. You guessed it; soups like vegetable or chicken noodle are great choices to develop your platform habit.

For a variety lunch, a salad and half sandwich make a good combination. And one step further, for a difference from time to time, eat a grilled chicken or grilled fish sandwich with no mayonnaise. And instead of French fries, ask for a plain baked potato. Do not put butter or sour cream on the potato, but you can sprinkle as much black pepper on it as you like and mix it together with your fork.

When you think about it, a bowl of non-cream-based soup and a salad make a great combination that leaves you full and satisfied. Another good option, if you want to feel full when you leave, is a vegetable plate.

As you can see, you can make many additions to your primary base platform of salads, but for your mind-set, think salads for lunch.

156

You will develop other personal favorites, but keep these two things in mind: (1) avoid fried foods, red meat, cheese and other dairy products, and (2) fruits and vegetables fill you up the most with the fewest calories possible.

Have a good lunch.

Dinner: Developing Variety

Dinner will depend, to a certain extent, on what you had for lunch. Vegetables are still your primary platform. A vegetable plate is easy to make at home or order in a restaurant.

Salad is a good choice for your evening meal, especially if you are in your weight-loss part of the plan. A dinner salad can also give you extra vegetables while allowing you to eat less of your entrée.

Pasta with sauce is a good addition on your dinner platform. With pasta, you are avoiding the saturated fat in meats and poultry, and you can come up with a large array of possibilities. You can also add fish or chicken as supplements to the pasta. But get in the habit of using tomato-based marinara sauce rather than the creamy cheese sauces commonly used at a restaurant and at home.

Another tier to the dinner platform is grilled fish or grilled chicken. You can choose how much and how often you will eat either as your main course. Chicken and fish both have some saturated fat in them but less than red meat. Grilled fish once or twice a week can be beneficial in helping you get certain omega-3s, which help in raising your HDL. Again, even if you have fish or chicken, vegetables and salad should be a significant part of the meal.

A nondairy-based soup makes a good addition. Have a cup with your salad, or eat a bowl as your entrée.

You can also have a veggie pizza with no cheese from time to time. I have one favorite I admit to indulging in occasionally: a small amount of grilled chicken with pineapple slices on a tomato base. By ordering a pizza with no cheese, you are leaving off the saturated fat.

Write down your primary basic platform for each meal and begin developing your basic eating strategy. Again, your platform foods will remain the same whether you are in a weight-loss phase or your ideal weight lifestyle of eating.

May you do as well as my friend did. It will be a great adventure.

11

Off-Limits Foods

Certain foods are completely off-limits. Set it in stone in your mind that you are going to eliminate some foods completely from your eating. Whenever you see them, you will turn and "run." No discussion. No thinking through.

These are your silent enemies:

- Cheese (If you order pizza, order it with vegetables only. They will make that at any pizza parlor.)
- Ice cream
- Salad dressing that is not fat-free
- Butter and margarine
- Whole milk (Use skim milk only.)
- Cookies and candy (No self-given rewards of sweets, and that includes Oreos.)
- Fried foods
- Chips that are not fat-free or baked
- Bacon and sausage

- Egg yolks (If you eat eggs, put them in an egg-white omelet with vegetables but no cheese.)
- Packaged snacks (Remember, fruit and nuts are your base snacks.)
- Cream-based sauces on chicken or fish, and cream-based soups (But you may sauté fish in olive oil.)

I tell you these off-limits foods for a reason. Unless you make a decision to avoid such foods, it is easy to let them creep back into your eating lifestyle. They can silently work on your arteries, with you being completely unaware of the damage. The Prescription for Life eating plan is the best prevention strategy you can have.

Otherwise, I am afraid you will end up like Bob.

Bob and I were classmates in medical school. He went into radiology and I went into surgery. We had kept in touch from time to time, and not many nights ago my wife and I happened to be visiting in a town near where he lived. I called and invited him and his wife to dinner to talk over old times.

It was the first time I had seen him in more than five years. He wasn't fat, but the lower part of his abdomen covered all but the bottom of his belt buckle. He was at least twenty pounds heavier than the last time I had seen him, and, overall, about thirty-five pounds overweight. And he walked funny. With each step, he had to flip each foot slightly upward before planting it on the sidewalk.

We discussed things we had done as we started our medical careers, about what our families had done the past few years, and about what happened to our doctor friends since those early days.

Then he told me about his foot drop. "It began just a couple of months ago. Every time I take a step, I have to sort of flip the end of my foot up before I put my foot down or my toes drag. They are not sure what is causing it, but, as I said, they are working me up for possible diabetes as the source."

I began asking him about his overall health, his cholesterol numbers, whether or not he exercised or had attempted to lose weight. We are friends, so this was more than just two doctors talking shop. I explained that if I had what he had and was told it was probably related to diabetes, I would do two things. First, I would get skinny. Next, I would exercise on the elliptical thirty minutes a day, five days a week, keeping my heart rate above 120 beats per minute.

That's when his wife chimed in. "He had three of his coronaries bypassed a few years ago. He isn't even mentioning that."

That shocked me. I realized his problems consisted of more than the possible diabetes affecting the nerves to his feet; they also included damaged arteries to his heart. Because of the arterial involvement, I added to the discussion a third lifestyle change: eating habits emphasizing fruits and vegetables, fish, whole grains, and nuts.

I told him that if I had what he had, I would be scared to death. (Actually, I told him three times.) I explained that I would get fanatical about changing my lifestyle. Scared to death, I told him again.

"I know my HDL Cholesterol is low, but I didn't know how to get it up," he said. With that acknowledgment, I smiled and told him he made a good lead-in statement. I then explained that the main way to elevate his HDL is to exercise and that weight loss is a close second. So he needed to do both.

He asked why I decided to lose weight. He had remembered me heavier during med school. I told him my "moment" story—the moment I tried on a pair of new trousers, realized I was going to have to increase the waist size for the third time, folded the pants and handed them back to the salesclerk, and made the decision to attain the ideal weight I had weighed in college.

That night, I told my old classmate and friend that this could be a "moment" time for him also. This could be the moment he decided to stop the progression of damage to his body in its tracks, right then. He could prevent any more plaque buildup in his arteries by controlling what he eats. He could control his diabetes by getting to an ideal weight. He could add numerous good, healthy years to his life.

He nodded his head in agreement.

Then I told him what had been on my mind ever since we began our after-dinner discussion at the restaurant. I explained to Bob that there was one concern I had that superseded all the others.

"What could happen to you would be much worse than foot drop. It could be much worse than another blockage to another artery in your heart. It could be worse than progression of your diabetes.

"You could have a stroke." I said it in almost a whisper. "The next time I see you, you could be having trouble making your words. I might not be able to understand what you are saying. You talk about having a foot drop now, but if you don't do something different with your lifestyle, later you may have such a limp that you have to use a walker. Or even worse, you may be in a wheelchair. The same blockages that are happening in the arteries of your heart are happening in the arteries of your brain. What scares me about your health is that you are sitting on a time bomb for a stroke. I guarantee you, Bob. It scares me to death to even imagine things like that happening to you."

I looked at him with all the sincerity I had in my heart for someone I had spent so much time with in medical school.

He quit nodding his head and said, "I realize what it's all about."

Before we parted company, I told him I would send him medical journal articles concerning the changes we had just discussed. As we parted, he gave me a hug that lasted longer than the usual good-bye clinch.

My greatest desire is for Bob to take all I said to heart.

I hope what scared me *to* death will scare him *from* death . . . for years to come.

I look forward to our next dinner. I want to see if he has placed certain foods completely off-limits. I want to see if he will turn and run from some of the food he had ordered for dinner. It will be great if I am unable to recognize the Bob I saw that night.

12

The Effects of Drinking Alcohol

There are a variety of diets out there. And most of them touch on the subject of alcohol.

So what about a glass of wine with your meal? It adds calories, but you may have read that it can help your heart by raising your HDL Cholesterol some. I will take a minute to give you the pros and cons on alcohol and diet and let you choose what you want.

In the medical literature concerning drinking alcohol, most articles say that if you do drink, you should drink in moderation. And most articles refer to moderation as up to one glass of wine a day for women and up to two drinks a day for men. Some add that men over sixty-five should also limit alcohol to one drink a day. The benefit given for drinking alcohol in moderation is that it can increase the good HDL Cholesterol.

But when you study such diets discussed in the medical literature, you will usually read that while alcohol in moderation may reduce the risk of blockage of your arteries in your heart, you should not start drinking if you don't already drink. Many articles point out the dangers alcohol can have on your body. Some studies even show that drinking purple grape juice may offer similar benefits for protecting your heart.

Ponder why the medical literature tells you not to begin drinking for the purpose of helping your arteries if you don't drink already. From strictly a medical standpoint, if something were better for your health than it was potentially bad for you, everyone would be encouraged to do it. If alcohol were a special pill that was proven to protect your arteries, the FDA would approve it and most everyone would be taking it. However, if the FDA found that pill could lead to significant detrimental health problems in a substantial number of people, the FDA governing board would pull it from the market. And soon you would see lawyers advertising on television stating that if something bad happened to you while you were on that particular pill you should call them in order to sue the company that produced the pill. No physician would be prescribing such a pill, especially if there were other, better ways to combat the problem.

Again, medically speaking, the best provision for raising your good HDL Cholesterol has been shown to be the combination of exercise and weight loss, not drinking alchohol.

An article in the *American Journal of Medicine* emphasizes the overall negative effect alcohol can have on your body. The researchers point out that alcohol can affect your blood pressure and weight negatively, as well as your tolerance to glucose. All these factors are detrimental to your arteries. On the other hand, exercise and weight control affect all three of these factors in a positive way. If you want to select the best possible program to protect your health, it makes more sense to concentrate on exercising and getting your weight to an ideal point.

Another article, in the *New England Journal of Medicine*, pointed out that there are serious health problems as well as social problems related to alcohol use. It said, for instance, that in a large population, any increase in alcohol consumption is associated with a proportionate increase in heavy drinking. It went on to point out that heavy drinking is a risk factor for strokes caused from bleeding or blockage of the arteries, as well as medical problems in other realms of your physical makeup. They concluded their study with the following statement: "Any public health recommendation that emphasizes the positive aspects of alcohol would be likely to do more harm than good."

Another interesting article related to alcohol consumption appeared in the World Cancer Research Fund and American Institute for Cancer Research latest write-up. They are one of the best authorities on cancer research, and they label causes of a particular cancer as being either "probable" or "convincing." For breast cancer in postmenopausal women, they point out that there is convincing evidence that alcohol increases the risk of breast cancer.

Another study shows the increased risk of breast cancer because of alcohol intake. In the *Nurses' Health Study*, 106,000 women were followed for more than twenty-five years. Women who had three to six drinks per week were 15 percent more likely to develop breast cancer than nondrinkers. It didn't matter what type of alcoholic beverage they drank. Of the women who averaged six to nineteen drinks per week, the increased risk for breast cancer was 20 percent. Now, for women who really liked their alcohol, this is what the study found. For those who drank more than nineteen drinks per week, the risk rose to a 50 percent increased risk for breast cancer.

Many studies on the relationship between alcohol and breast cancer mostly blamed heavy drinking, but a new study in the *Journal of the American Medical Association* found that light to moderate drinkers also face an increased risk of breast cancer.

Heavy alcohol consumption carries many health problems with it. As a Mayo Clinic special report article states, from a medical standpoint, "If you don't already drink . . . don't start."

You now know what your primary food platform should be for breakfast, lunch, and dinner, and even the pros and cons of alcohol. Next we move to the lifestyle that affects your weight. You will find this information helpful whether you are obese or presently at your ideal weight. Learn why weight control is so important.

Part 3

Reach Your Ideal Weight

Nothing good ever comes from being overweight. Are you at your ideal weight? Do you even know what your ideal weight is? Are you in the small elite group of 12 percent of Americans who are at their ideal weight? Do you know the harm you bring to your body by being overweight?

You are about to get a good insight concerning the dangers that come with being overweight and how to achieve and maintain your ideal weight for the rest of your life. You will avoid fad diets because you will learn how few people are able to remain at their goal weight once they reach it with such a diet. There are numerous diet plans to try, but you want one that is sustainable. You want to acquire knowledge about a weight-loss plan that is based on what is medically healthy. You are about to learn some secrets that will help you get there and some rules to adopt to keep you there—from now on, for the remainder of your life.

Losing weight is not about dieting—it's all about developing the proper lifestyle.

13

Determining Your
Ideal Weight

Being overweight is a statement of relativity. You should read this section whether you are at your ideal weight or two hundred pounds over. The information here will make you aware of how important weight is in keeping your body machine functioning at optimum efficiency. One of the most significant things you can ever do for yourself is to maintain an ideal weight. It is no shame to be overweight. The shame comes when you *stay* overweight.

Good to Remember

Need to lose weight? Fruits and vegetables contain the least number of calories for a given portion size. Fiber makes you feel full on fewer calories. You don't need to count the calories; count the foods that give you the least calories.

Your Ideal Weight Matters

Your primary goal in the Prescription for Life plan lifestyle is reaching your *ideal weight*.

If you are fifty pounds overweight, pay attention.
If you are five pounds overweight, pay attention.
If you are at your ideal weight, pay attention.

Because even at your ideal weight, some days you are going to fluctuate upward, and you will need to automatically switch to your weight-loss mode for twenty-four to forty-eight hours to get back to your ideal weight.

The Prescription for Life plan focuses on eating properly while losing your excess weight and then staying at your optimal weight permanently. You are trying to drop pounds the quickest way possible but also learning how to develop a lifestyle of eating the proper foods. You will lose weight, and at the same time you will be developing your healthy eating habits. You will replace your old eating habits with proper ones that you will have the rest of your life.

His friends called him Wilson. He reminded me of the parable in the Bible about putting new wine into old wineskins. The message of that parable is if you put new wine in old wineskins, the new wine could cause the old wineskin to burst. The application for us is if you change your life for a better, new one, don't ever try to take your newfound lifestyle back to your old ways of doing things.

Wilson was nearly one hundred pounds overweight when he decided to start a diet that had been successful in taking pounds off a friend at work. "It worked great. I saw it happen myself. I couldn't believe it," was the way he described watching his friend lose weight. He ordered the food he was to eat. In addition to that he made smoothies for certain meals, and then if he were to eat out, his meal would consist of only protein. He was faithful to the plan. He dropped every pound he had set his goal to do.

But then he did something that happens to the majority of people who go on such fad diets. Once they have successfully reached their goal, they return to their old habits. Once the mail-order food quit coming, once Wilson had completed the course, once he thought he was successful, he took his new wine and poured it into his old wineskin. He slowly went back to eating the same foods he had been addicted to for so many years.

The last time I had seen him he was trim, and smiling, and talking to everyone in his office. Even his pants were non-pleated and ironed. But that was a little over a year ago. This time I could not believe my eyes. He had regained his weight. Maybe more. There certainly was no smile, and he barely looked up when I walked into the room. He just stayed hunched over his computer. I couldn't bring myself to ask him about it.

Wilson obviously didn't know about the old wineskin story. He didn't realize that if he lost weight using one strategy for eating but returned to his old lifestyle with food, he would regain his weight. Poor Wilson could have developed a strategy for eating that would not only ensure losing weight but also guarantee that he could continue the same way of eating without regaining the weight.

Once he had won the battle, it was just too easy for him to go back to his old eating habits.

Say No to Fad Diets

You probably have been on some type of fad diet sometime in the past. There are two problems with such programs. Many of them have a harmful effect on your arteries, and the vast majority of them result in you eventually regaining your weight. Why? Because you return to your former eating habits once your ideal weight is reached. The Prescription for Life plan diet is different. The eating habits you learn while you are losing weight are the same ones you will continue once you reach your optimal weight.

With the Prescription for Life plan, your desires for certain tastes and foods will change. You won't want to go back to the harmful foods you used to enjoy, like Wilson did. There will be a smooth transition from the weight-loss phase of the plan to the lifetime strategy. Never forget: the whole weight-loss process of any diet is a complete failure if you regain weight. Your goal is about good health and a better quality of life—up to the end.

Exercise

There is a lot more to losing weight than just dieting. The majority of diet programs leave out or miss the mark on that fact. *Exercise* is a key factor to your overall success. The Prescription for Life plan is not about food alone. To understand permanent ideal weight, you have to understand the significance of exercise in preventing the aging process.

I like to use the simple example of a Brown University study, where two groups of overweight women were compared. One group dieted and exercised while the other group only dieted. The group that dieted *and* exercised lost almost twice the weight than the ones who did not exercise. Those numbers make a loud statement concerning the significance of exercise. It is another one of those "walking-around-sense" realizations. If you want to lose weight and keep it off, do more than just diet.

You do burn up some calories when you exercise, but losing weight is a lot more than just burning calories. A rule of thumb number is that you expend about a hundred calories per mile.

That is whether you are walking or running. But it was not just the calories that caused the group of women who dieted plus exercised to lose almost twice the weight of those who did not exercise. A lot more happens to your body when you exercise. It's almost magical. We will discuss that fact in more detail when we get to the exercise portion of the study, but right now, I want you to set in your mind the significance exercise has on losing weight. I will let you decide whether you are going to be walking at a fast pace or jogging an eight-minute mile, but you will be exercising in this weight-loss program.

A Plan That Works

I had known her about eight years when she asked me about losing weight. She had tried so many ways to get the pounds off but "just couldn't make it happen," she said. She is a caretaker and one of the friendliest ladies you would ever meet. She would not be labeled obese, but she was significantly overweight. She had diabetes and high blood pressure. After being carried to the emergency room by ambulance one night because of her diabetes, she inquired about what she could do to lose weight and protect her health. "I want to be around for my children and grandchildren," she told me.

I explained the basics of the Prescription for Life plan and asked her if she had ever exercised as a part of any of her weight-loss programs. She laughed as she shook her head no. After I explained to her the importance of exercise in conjunction with dieting, she began jogging on a treadmill five days a week. She had made the decision to begin the journey.

That was over a year ago, and now she is off half of the medications she was on. She cooks completely differently. She continues on the treadmill five days a week, and she has trimmed down so much that her close girlfriends make fun of her for not having a large enough behind. That is the best compliment anyone can get, especially when she remembers the night she rode to the hospital in the ambulance.

How to Figure Your Ideal Weight

The Prescription for Life plan calls for you to sustain your ideal weight. The question most people ask is how they can know what their ideal weight is supposed to be. There are many ways to figure what someone your particular age, or height, or body build should weigh, but when you get down to it, you will decide, and I won't argue with you. There are average body weight tables you can find that give some idea, but you have to realize that the so-called *average* weight is probably too high for what you want to shoot for because so many Americans are overweight to begin with.

So we are left with another formula called BMI, or body mass index. It goes like this if you want to figure yours.

$$BMI = \frac{weight\ in\ pounds\ x\ 703}{height\ in\ inches,\ squared}$$

BMI gives you a specific number that you can calculate to see if you are overweight. The problem is that it doesn't give you a specific ideal weight. Anything over 30 is considered obese, between 25 and 30 is called overweight, and if you are below 25, that is considered a normal weight.

In general, one-third of Americans fall into the normal BMI category, one-third into the overweight group, and the other third into the obese classification. You may feel comfortable with your present weight because you are in the "normal" BMI category. But you still need to pay attention because the one-third of individuals who are in the normal group do fall into the overweight category intermittently.

You have to keep in mind that even if you fall into the "normal" category, you may not be at your ideal weight. Only about a third of the people in the normal weight group are at their ideal weight, and less than 12 percent of Americans are at their ideal weight. In figuring your BMI, you definitely want to be within the normal range of below 25. But that is only a starting point. You must remember that there can be a huge difference between "normal weight," as defined by BMI, and your true "ideal weight." Let me give you an example.

I had a friend who had a significant pouch at the bottom of his abdomen. (He thought he looked great for his age.) We were in the gym when he informed me that his doctor had told him he was at his ideal weight. I asked him how he knew his ideal weight, and he responded, "Because my BMI was in the normal range." I looked at him with my head cocked. There he was, in the gym, exercise shirt bulging out over the bottom of his abdomen, bragging that he was at his ideal weight. He had no idea about the difference between "normal weight" with the BMI scale and "ideal weight."

He saw me looking at him with my head tilted and asked what was wrong with what he said. I explained that his BMI wasn't the same as ideal weight.

"If being in the normal BMI range isn't my ideal weight, how do I know what my ideal weight is?" he responded.

"Turn sideways and look in the mirror," was my spontaneous reply. "Just look at your belly."

As he turned his head down to look at the protrusion, I explained that what was sticking out was an apron of fat tissue just on the inside of the front part of his lower abdomen. That apron is the favorite spot for the body to store extra fat. "If you look pretty trim everywhere except your abdomen, it is your internal fatty apron that will disappear if you lose weight." I realized I had gotten the point across when he placed both hands on this lower abdomen and smiled.

In essence, BMI numbers are good to use if you are dividing individuals into categories of being normal, overweight, and obese—but BMI is not what you use to determine your ideal weight. You first get into that normal column, then turn sideways and look in the mirror. If the image in the mirror doesn't look the way you want it to, then you are not at your ideal weight. Your personal ideal weight is not determined by some specific scale; it is decided by you (after looking in the mirror about a hundred times).

You can also get numbers concerning limits on waist circumferences or abdominal fat measurements or a sundry of other ideas to determine whether you are overweight. Some go back to their high school weight or college weight and decide that is the weight they want to return to. If you were healthy when you were younger, that may help you in deciding. Others decide ideal weight depending on their particular body build.

There is another formula a little more specific than BMI that shoots pretty lean but may also give you an idea of what to go for. I sort of like this one, but still, you have to decide for yourself the goal weight you want. I just encourage you to go to the leanest number that comes to your mind.

Here is the second formula, and it is related just to your height. It is strict but gives the best idea of what to aim for when figuring ideal weight. This second formula aims low, but there is nothing wrong with using these numbers as an initial consideration. For men, use 105 pounds as baseline for the first five feet of your height, then add five pounds to that baseline for every inch over five feet. For women, use ninety-five pounds as baseline for the first five feet, then add four pounds for every inch over five feet. Again, this gives you an approximate ideal weight, but you will have to fine-tune it for your body build.

A friend of mine gives good advice on deciding your goal weight. He was 220 pounds and did the figuring on height and several other formulas and came up with an optimal weight of 185. But when he got to 185, he said it didn't feel right and ended up at 175, where he felt the healthiest. That has been his weight for the past five years. He says he will easily keep that weight from now on. Figure what goal you want to set for your ideal weight and go for it. The only advice I give you is to go for low. (You can always add a few pounds back on if you end up weighing too little.)

I was asked recently if medical science has come up with a way to help prevent cancer. I replied, "No one has developed a magic pill, but there has been a significant finding concerning what you are asking." I gave him a statement from the World Cancer Research Fund and the American Institute for Cancer Research. They found that about a third of cancers in the United States could be prevented with lifestyle changes to develop a "healthy diet, regular physical activity, and maintaining a healthy weight." That is another one of those "walking-around-sense" bits of information. This is an organization whose sole purpose is finding ways to prevent cancer.

Personally, if they point out that I can reduce my chances of developing one of the more common cancers by a third—by eating the proper foods, exercising, and maintaining an ideal weight—I am going to figure my ideal weight and get to it as fast as I can. Think about it. What better insurance policy could you possibly obtain? You shouldn't have to do anything but look at yourself in the mirror to make a decision as simple as that one.

The weight-loss part of the Prescription for Life plan is an ongoing process—getting to your ideal weight and remaining there. A good aid in this process is weighing yourself every morning. If you find yourself a pound over your ideal weight, shift your eating strategy from your normal eating habits to the weight-loss style until you are back at your ideal weight. That may take just a day, or it might take several. You control your ideal weight by closely monitoring what you weigh.

Some tell me they do not weigh themselves but rather go by waist size. If you go by such a plan, just keep in mind that by the time you realize you are one inch larger in waist size, it will take you a much longer period to regain your ideal weight.

Whether you are a pound or fifty pounds overweight, it's all relative and all proportional. So now let's look at how extra weight harms your body.

14

The Penalty for Being Overweight

There is a direct correlation between body weight and premature mortality.

That is another "walking-around-sense" factor for you to acknowledge. The more overweight you are, the greater your chances of an early death. Just let that sink into your head, and you will begin understanding why you should be shooting for an optimal goal weight.

Do you remember the gentleman I mentioned who went to the nursing home and saw there were no obese patients there? "They were already dead," he said.

Most people begin to gain several pounds a year in early midlife and, before long, add twenty, thirty, or more pounds without giving it a thought. You become accustomed to that extra fat around your waist because everyone else your age has it. Then one day you realize you have had to increase your pants' waist size by several inches. You didn't think too much of it, but now you know that adding those extra pounds is significantly increasing your odds of developing high blood pressure, diabetes, and heart disease. You don't want to increase those odds, especially since you are only twenty or forty pounds overweight and have never even thought about the health consequence of that extra weight. The truth is that if you understand the damage you are doing to your body, you most likely will do something about it.

If I asked a hundred people if they think smoking lowers a smoker's life expectancy, probably 99 percent would agree that it does. Yes, I have talked to individuals who still don't believe smoking causes lung cancer, but almost everyone knows the dangers of smoking. You know if you smoke you are cutting years off your life, not to mention the quality of the years you do live. I don't think anyone would argue that point. Medical statistics prove these ideas.

So let's compare these negatives of smoking with the negatives of being overweight. Is being overweight just as bad for your health as smoking is?

Let's start with the effect each has on longevity. In one of the leading medical journals, the *Annals of Internal Medicine*, an interesting report does such a comparison. It states that being overweight and obesity in adulthood are definitely linked to an increased risk for death, as well as an increased risk for disease. They compared a normal weight group with an obese group to find the life expectancy of each group. They found that obesity results in 5.8 years loss of life expectancy for males and 7.1 years for females. You talk about throwing away years, being overweight or obese does just that. The next time you see an obese individual walking around the mall, remind yourself that their extra weight is costing them six to seven years of their life.

Keep in mind that we are comparing being overweight with smoking, as each relates to your health. So here is the tie-in, the big point in the research mentioned above: the decreases in life expectancy of being overweight are similar to those seen with smoking. Let's look at the perils of smoking so you can put being overweight and obese in proper perspective. Here's what the American Cancer Society has to say: "Half of all those who continue to smoke will die from smoking-related diseases."

That statement makes you wonder why anyone in the whole wide world would continue smoking, doesn't it? However, don't be too critical, because in a few minutes you may wonder why in the world anyone would continue being overweight.

Another statement: smoking accounts for at least 30 percent of all cancer deaths and 87 percent of lung cancer deaths. That statement also makes you wonder why someone who smokes wouldn't do something to take care of that danger. Could being overweight be a comparable danger?

One last fact about smoking: smoking is a major cause of heart disease and cerebrovascular disease—strokes. That statement is talking directly about the arteries of the heart and brain. It would make "walking-around-sense" to quit smoking, wouldn't it? It is very easy to think someone ought to do everything they can to quit smoking after knowing all those facts. But do you think it would make similar sense to get to an ideal weight if you read studies showing that being overweight and obese is similar to the hazards of smoking?

If you can realize how bad smoking is for someone else's body, why not acknowledge that being overweight and obese is just as bad for your body—and wake up and do something about it?

Obesity *lowers* the "hero" HDL Cholesterol by 20 to 30 percent

This statement is eye-catching, especially after learning how important HDL Cholesterol is in protecting your arteries and preventing the aging process from occurring. Obesity lowers your good cholesterol by 20 to 30 percent. When you take that figure to heart, the Prescription for Life plan becomes easier and easier to follow. But the story gets even worse:

Obesity can *raise* the "lethal" LDL Cholesterol by as much as 50 percent

The bottom line is that you don't want to carry any excess weight around on your body. So how do you shed those extra pounds and keep them off?

15

Weight Loss 101

Being overweight is not a *simple* problem—it is a *major* problem. Most people who are overweight are concerned about their appearance. Very few look at the medical implications on their body. So many studies in the medical literature show that extra weight leads to a much earlier death than if one is at an ideal weight. One such study reported a direct correlation between body weight and mortality—that the rate of mortality increased *progressively* with more weight added. The damage doesn't happen suddenly when you reach one hundred pounds overweight; it progresses one pound at a time, beginning with that initial pound.

We look at ourselves every day, but seldom do we stand there and say, "I am in the process of slowly killing myself and not doing anything about it." If there were a stranger standing beside you with a gun, and you knew that person would shoot you sometime in the future, you would call the police and get rid of him. Some may appease themselves by saying they are overweight but not obese. The difference between the two is only degrees of damage to their arteries.

Forget how you look. Stop worrying about your appearance. Put your excess weight in proper perspective. Begin thinking how much longer and more actively you can live if you lose the extra weight.

How to Achieve and Maintain Your Ideal Weight

Diet and exercise *together* are what make it all happen—losing excess weight and maintaining your ideal weight. The vast majority who desire to lose weight and keep it off attempt it by diet alone. Diet by itself very seldom works for sustained weight loss. Don't go there. Forget it. Burn every article, every book that has a special diet plan for you to attempt. You may lose some weight, but you won't keep it off once you complete that particular cycle of eating. A report in the National Weight Control Registry states that only 2 to 20 percent of dieters are able to maintain their weight loss. Would you buy into a stock that gives you only a 20 percent chance of making a profit? Would you take a medication from your doctor if she told you it works only 2 percent of the time?

You need a lifestyle strategy, not a weight-loss plan.

The sad thing is that so many who lose their excess weight regain it. And if they adopt a quick-fix fad diet plan, 95 percent of the ones who do lose weight not only regain it but also add more pounds to it within a three-year period.

Let me make a point with you about the dangers of losing weight and then regaining it. It is worse, health-wise, to lose weight and then put it back on than it is to never lose the weight in the first place. Very few people realize this physiological danger in losing weight and regaining it. Very seldom will you look in the mirror and think that you need to do something to protect your arteries to prevent aging. No, you just think you will look better if you lose some weight.

Let's say you lose down to your ideal weight by changing your eating habits drastically for a period of time. Then what? It's like getting accepted to medical school and, once there, wondering what you need to do to stay in school.

On a typical fad diet, people lose weight, then regain it all in three years. Guess what you are doing to your arteries as you regain all that weight. As you add those forty pounds, you are igniting LDL Cholesterol damage to your arterial walls with every pound you are regaining. It's simple mathematics. It would be better if you had never lost the weight in the first place. Don't compound the problem. Don't put your arteries through all those battles again.

Your weight-loss plan needs to do three things to be successful. One, it has to help you lose weight. Two, it must enhance good health. And three, it has to be permanent.

Eat the Best Foods with the Fewest Calories

Should you keep track of the number of calories you take in? The answer is yes and no. Calories are important in one sense. The more you take in, the more ounces you put on . . . and the more calories you burn, the fewer ounces you will weigh.

When deciding which foods you are going to eat, it's good for you to know a little fact we learned early in medical school: a gram of fat contains nine calories while a gram of sugar or protein contains only four calories. So if you are eating something fried rather than grilled, you are adding numerous calories to the food. Don't go to the trouble of trying to count how many more calories French fries are going to contain versus the same potato baked. Just realize the fries are going to contain more calories than the baked potato, plus they are probably going to be fried in oil high in saturated fat that is going to elevate your LDL in addition to adding calories. In the end, it's easier to learn which foods to eat rather than adding up your calories.

The main foods that satisfy hunger with the fewest calories are fruits and vegetables. Weight Watchers gives a great insight into the importance of these two food groups for losing excess weight.

As I pointed out earlier, Weight Watchers is based on a point system that includes calorie content of a food. It has been one of the most successful weight-loss programs. But Weight Watchers recently changed their point system. You can eat as many fruits and vegetables as you want without having to count the points. By this, they are encouraging their clients to eat foods that will fill their stomachs, satisfy their appetites, are of good nutrition, and have a low calorie count. Fruits and vegetables form a significant basis for your new eating lifestyle. You will be surprised how you will satisfy your hunger by having all the fruits and vegetables you want as your primary source of calories.

Here's a quick story about a college football coach friend of mine. One day he mentioned, "I have decided to lose twenty pounds." He said it directly and without a doubt, with all the authority that goes along with being a coach. He didn't look all that much overweight, but he was pudgy (if you know what I mean). Anyway, he asked for the best way to lose it the quickest. I knew he was wired in such a way that once he made up his mind, he would do it. I spent maybe five minutes explaining the idea that fruits and vegetables would fill him up and that if he disciplined himself to stick to these foods as his primary diet, he would lose weight.

Normally, if you walked into his office any day of the week, you would have seen homemade cakes, plates of brownies, and cookies of all sorts that fans brought by for all the coaches to eat. I told him, "All that must go." He said, "No problem."

Then we went over a baseline Prescription for Life plan for each meal, emphasizing fruits and vegetables, and he listened intently. I then told him he would eat nothing between meals or after dinner. He answered again, "No problem." That's all I told him.

I was by his office one evening two weeks later, and he matter-of-factly told me he had lost nine pounds. He said it wasn't any trouble. He had taken all the tempting foods, cakes, cookies, and the like out of his office and put them in the conference room where all the coaches met. He told me to wait right where I was while he went to the conference room and brought back a plate that had four brownies on it. He held them out toward me and said, "I never even wanted to sample one of these things." I smiled because I really liked the way he was humbly bragging. He said he never got hungry.

That little story was told to whet your appetite for fruits and vegetables. You can get into debates about which fruits and which vegetables are better than others, but I like to keep it simple. Most of the people I talk to are like that football coach. He is changing from the juiciest hamburger, crispiest French fry, and creamiest ice cream diet you can imagine to a simple one focused on fruits and vegetables.

I didn't want to make things complex. I didn't want to tell him tuna and salmon are better than whatever other fish he likes to eat. Just getting him off the barbecue pork he was eating two nights a week and eating any kind of fish is a huge lifestyle change for him.

It can be for you too.

The Effect of Weight on the Heart

There is a direct correlation between being overweight and dying from heart disease. One such report was done in Kentucky, where they studied almost three thousand autopsies to determine the correlation between being overweight and dying of heart disease. This was not a study of LDL Cholesterol or a study of whether the person ate red meat, or fried foods, or fatty desserts—or fruits and vegetables—or exercised.

This was primarily a study to see how many of the people who died a natural death had blockages in the arteries of their heart and what percent of those individuals were overweight. It was a simple study that we can all comprehend, and here is what they found.

Of the ones who died from heart disease, 71 percent had an unhealthy BMI. From this you can extrapolate that if someone is overweight, you don't have to know all his or her numbers for cholesterol, or blood pressure, or diabetes level. You can look at being overweight as being the primary factor in determining that your body is unhealthy and that you stand a greater risk for having disease in the arteries of your heart and brain. Being overweight, in itself, is deadly. If you are overweight, the odds are against you. (Remember, go to the nursing home and you will see mostly skinny people.)

You don't need to be a doctor to understand this. The physiological reality is that being overweight puts a strain on your heart. Having that extra ten pounds or extra fifty pounds of fat on your body means your heart has to pump more blood to that extra tissue to keep it alive. Your heart has to work harder.

As your excess unhealthy tissue increases, the volume of blood in your body also has to increase. Your heart pumps this extra blood through a network of newly formed tiny arteries and even smaller capillaries. In turn, the heart has to generate higher pressures to overcome this sieve effect the heart pumps the blood through. You can imagine the strain this puts on the pumping action of the heart. There is no auxiliary pump your heart can call on for help. It just has to do more work on its own.

Finally, it gets to a point when it can't pump the blood effectively and the pump begins to fail, just unable to take care of all the extra work. You begin to accumulate fluid in your ankles because the pump is not efficient enough to pump all the fluid. Next, this extra fluid begins to accumulate in your lungs, and you become short of breath—and if you don't wake up and take control of your body, your pump eventually will fail.

Your death certificate will read: *cardiac failure.* But it ought to read: *failure to comply with owner's manual.* Take control of your weight. Don't ignore reality.

Take control of your life. On vacation a year ago, my wife and I were at a dinner with two other couples. One of the men was at least fifty pounds overweight and had been for over fifteen years. He informed us he had high blood pressure and had been on medication for it for almost ten years. He said his doctor had told him if he lost weight, he could come off his blood pressure medicine. "But I like to eat too much to lose the amount of weight to get my blood pressure down." He laughed, almost defiantly. "I would rather just take the medicine." He didn't lose a second getting the next bite into his mouth. He had no idea I knew anything about being overweight causing high blood pressure. He did not know that I already knew his future, even though I had only just met him.

My thoughts about him went something like this. I wondered, as he talked about his children, if he had the slightest idea that he was not going to be around for them as long as he could. I wondered if he realized how less active he was going to become as time went on. And I wondered why in the world he would not take his doctor's advice about losing weight and taking care of his blood pressure.

High blood pressure is only a small part of his picture, especially in the days to come.

Next will be his blood sugar. It will begin to creep up. And his doctor will tell him that if he loses weight, he won't have to take medication for his elevated blood sugar—or he will have to take a pill to try to control it. He'll take the pill.

Next . . . and he has no idea, plus he wouldn't listen even if I told him . . . will be the walls of his arteries throughout his body. The sugar will begin to wear on the lining of his arteries. And his blood pressure will continue to pound the LDL splinters into his arteries. He will become impotent. And he will eventually block the blood flow of oxygen needed for his heart pump to keep working.

Of course, he believes medication is the answer, not prevention. (The vast majority of Americans believe the same.) Even if I told him differently, he thinks his medication will make his blood pressure perfect and his sugar medication will take care of his elevated sugar. He is the type who believes that medication is equally as good as the natural body in keeping all this in check. He actually believes that man-made medication is equal to the thousands of natural body checks the human body has built in to keep it working properly. Unfortunately, he is not alone. Most other people also think this way.

He has no idea. He is not the kind to listen. So I didn't bother telling him that his doctor was right—he ought to lose to an ideal weight. I didn't bother telling him that he is going to end up being one of the 50 percent of Americans who will die from disease in their heart and brain arteries. I didn't even ask him if he had ever thought seriously about losing weight. I didn't mention anything about what he might do to improve his aging process.

Later that night, I kept thinking that he represents so many people who simply don't know. I kept thinking that I wished I could discover something to wake up such people and get them to commit. I was wishing I could get him interested in the Prescription for Life plan. I even told my wife that night after we got home that he was the type of person you would be wasting your time on discussing weight loss or lifestyle change.

Now you won't believe the rest of this story. I told you there were two couples with us at diner. Well, after my wife and I left, the other couple explained to the overweight gentleman who I was and that I could help him with his weight problem. I got a phone call the next morning from him, asking if I would mind spending some time to discuss how to develop a new lifestyle. For some reason, he had come to one of those *moments* in life when he suddenly realized the need to do something about taking care of his body.

The following evening, we sat on a porch, discussing his situation.

"How overweight do you think you are?"

"I don't know exactly, but a lot," he explained.

"What would be your plan to get the extra weight off?"

He shrugged his shoulders and said he would not eat as much. But when I pressed him to explain a strategy, he couldn't.

"What are your hopes?" I asked. "Where do you see yourself in five years? In ten years?" He wanted to have a normal life, he said. He wanted to be there for his wife and grandchildren and to be active as he got older. He didn't want to get old before his time, he said.

I spent considerable time going over the basics of the Prescription for Life plan, and I am not sure I have seen anyone get as excited as he did. During that week of vacation, he completely changed his lifestyle of eating, exercising, and starting toward his ideal weight. After our vacation was over, I would wonder from time to time if he had been successful. I felt wholeheartedly that he had made the commitment, but still, I didn't know for sure.

One year later I met him again at the same vacation spot. I hardly recognized him. "How much have you lost?" He told me he'd lost sixty-four pounds and said, "I want advice about getting the last forty off." And he wanted to know now how to prepare for how he will eat then. "Because that day is coming," was his near gleeful statement.

It is so encouraging to work with someone who sees the light. Who wakes up to the reality of what they are doing to their body. And especially to see them set the goal and commitment to make it happen. This gentleman is wired like that—in his business, in his marriage, in most of what he does in life. He will never again say that he will "just take the medicine" rather than take the action to control the problem. He is another real encouragement for you to decide the best course to travel and get started on it.

16

Weight Loss Secrets
and Easy Steps

Write down your goal weight—your ideal weight. Make a commitment to reach it. Put it on a yellow Post-it note and stick it on your mirror. Carry it with you in your purse, in your wallet. Write it down—you can reach it.

This chapter is for everyone, whether you need to lose weight or maintain your present weight. It is divided into two sections, "secrets" and "easy steps." You are going to learn how to use these secrets and easy steps to maintain your lifestyle.

Three Secrets for Losing Weight

1. Eat Vegetables and Fruits

The first secret is to fill up on vegetables and fruits. Has anyone ever told you the secret to losing weight is to eat as much as you want? Well, that's exactly what you can do—with fruits and vegetables, that is. There will be no limit to the amount of fruits and vegetables you eat because of two facts. One is that both foods have lots of fiber and will give you a full sensation, which will take away your desire to eat more. And second, vegetables and fruits have the fewest calories for the amount of food you consume. Your first secret to losing weight is to develop eating habits that center around getting full with the fewest calories.

I know what you may be thinking: "He is going to ask me to eat mostly . . . what?" It may not sound very appetizing, but after you incorporate this secret into your strategy for eating, it will surprise you how you become accustomed to having vegetables as a basis of your meal rather than meat. Plus, over time, your desire for the foods you think will be impossible to give up right now will decline greatly. Your desire for a thick, juicy steak will drift out of the "urgent" part of your brain. If you don't believe me now, I just ask you to try this for eight weeks and watch it happen. You are addicted to the foods you enjoy so much. You can change that addiction to something healthier. Don't argue. Just try it.

2. Be Mindful of Portions

Portions fall into two categories. When you eat out, whatever portion that particular restaurant presents is the portion you have to deal with. When you eat at home, you have the choice of what you place on your plate. Home is much easier to control than restaurants. At home, you simply tell yourself that you are going to place a small portion on your plate, sit down, and enjoy your meal. That situation is controllable, especially if you practice the ten-minute factor and tell yourself that, for now, this is what you are going to place on your plate—and that is all you eat.

But problems come when you eat out. You order at a restaurant and are given a huge serving of everything. So what do you do?

If you're eating with your spouse or a friend, and the two of you can agree on a particular entrée, you can order a kitchen split. You will be given a half portion of the fish or chicken order, plus a full order of the vegetables. You can add a soup or salad and end up with an abundance of food to eat. Or they will simply split the entrée in half and serve it on two separate plates.

If you're eating alone, you can simply ask that the kitchen place half of the meal into a take-home container. That way you have something to eat at home for lunch or dinner the next day, or you place it in your refrigerator and find it there a week later and end up throwing it away. That's okay too—it's better than eating it all at that initial evening. Some restaurants will even let you order a half portion. The charge will be a little more than half price, but at least you aren't getting the entire large amount.

A third way of ordering less if you're eating alone is to order from the appetizer menu and add a couple of vegetables on the side. That's all you will need if you are in weight-losing mode. Don't get trapped thinking you are eating well with just an appetizer if that starter food is fried, battered, and cheese covered. So many times they are, but many times you will see smoked tuna or salmon, or a small skewer of grilled shrimp, or similar food found in the entrée section of the menu. Plus, you can add soup or salad to your appetizer if you are really hungry and end up with a satisfying meal. Don't overlook this option. Most of the time you will get plenty to eat if you follow this platform. A salad and appetizer is not a bad combination.

The fourth and final way, which is almost impossible when you remind yourself that you are paying for the entire amount of food, is to simply leave food on your plate. If you end up in this situation, at least give it the best try you can. Visually divide the plate into what you will and won't eat. Once you have eaten what you decided to eat, activate the ten-minute factor and stop eating for ten minutes while you order a cup of coffee and sit and talk with your friends. That way you can return to your food if you are still hungry ten minutes later. But I assure you, nine times out of ten, you won't eat another bite because by that time, the "I'm full" signal will have started flashing and you will realize that your main goal is to lose weight rather than to clean your plate (like your mother taught you).

By the way, if you are eating with friends, look at the mealtime as just that—time with friends. Center your attention on being with them, talking with them, enjoying them. Make them the central theme rather than your food. You will eat slower, talk more, and before long, you are not so hungry.

3. Don't Eat Snacks

The third secret is no snacks. Listen to this next statement: controlling your snacking is one of the most significant aspects of weight loss. People add many surplus calories, resulting in extra weight, because of "just a light afternoon snack" or "just a bite of something before going to bed." You do not realize all the extra nonproductive calories you are adding each time you snack. Don't fool yourself into thinking you will eat less at mealtime if you snack between meals. Don't get trapped into thinking snack calories subtract from meal calories. You pat yourself on the back for not eating a dessert at supper last night, but it doesn't click in your mind that you can put on as many or more calories with a snack as you can with the dessert.

Begin at home and in your office by removing the snack temptations that most Americans go for. Walk through an office building and look. The majority of overweight people have some type of food sitting on their desk. I can't stress it enough. Remove the temptation. Remove the junk. Remove them from your cupboard, fridge, shelves, and office. Don't let your eyes even have to glance at them when you open a cabinet or drawer. Such a big part of temptation is sight. Get the snacks out of the way and out of your vision.

Relax. It's not that you will never eat another snack in your life. Once at your goal weight, you will eat snacks, but first you will develop the habit of eating nuts and fruits. (More on that later.)

Now that you know the significance of eating fruits and vegetables, controlling portion size, and not eating snacks between meals, let's look at some basic rules concerning what you eat at mealtimes. I call these basics "easy steps" for weight loss.

Eight Easy Steps for Controlling Weight

1. Food Focus versus Calorie Focus

Many diets emphasize calories. Calories are indeed significant because your body runs on calories. You take x number in, and it takes x number to run the ship. The calories not used are stored as fat in your body. It doesn't take much of a medical mind to realize that if you continue taking in more calories than you burn, you gain weight. So calories are significant, but you are not going to count them. You are going to learn which foods contain the fewest calories and eat more of those foods. You count the foods rather than the calories.

Fatty foods have more calories than nonfatty foods. As you already know, fat has over twice the calories, ounce for ounce, as protein or sugar. If you fry something, you will be adding about a third more calories. Again, it doesn't take much intelligence to realize that when someone eats fatty meals or desserts, they are taking in many more calories than with foods such as fruits and vegetables. Many fad diets will have you eating something that may be fewer calories than another food, but the lower calorie food may contain a multitude of saturated fat or dietary cholesterol that skyrocket your LDL Cholesterol. In such cases, the saturated fat factor is much more important than the number of calories the particular food may contain. Don't get hung up on the number of calories; rather, get focused on the aging potential of a particular food.

2. Snacks

Once you have reached your goal weight, you will be able to eat snacks. Develop the habit of utilizing fruits or nuts as your snack foods. Even though they are snacks, the foods will be healthy. I remind you here that there will be days when you realize you are a pound or two above your goal weight. That is the day you go back to your "no snacks" rule until you are back on your set course.

3. No Bread before Meals

Whole-grain breads do not have saturated fat, which is good. But they do contain calories. Think of breads as sugar. Most people can relate sugar to extra calories, and that is basically what that bread represents—extra calories. During the weight-loss part of your plan, the less bread, the better. Don't dive into that basket of bread that appears on your table. Once you see the food you ordered, you immediately realize how much better that food will taste, calorie for calorie, than the bread.

Try this: the next time you are in a restaurant where they bring you a basket of bread, hold off eating it until after you have completed your main course. Then after your meal, see if you want some of the bread sitting there in the basket. I'll bet nine times out of ten you will not wolf down the bread like you would have when they first set it before you. Taking in those premeal bread calories is completely preventable. Even after reaching your ideal weight, you can have your toast for breakfast and half sandwich for lunch, but no extra-calorie bread before your meal is still a good habit to have developed.

4. No Desserts

This step is difficult but important. Enjoy the company of your friends while they eat their dessert and you have your coffee or tea or just chat. If you are losing weight, no dessert after your meal is on your primary platform strategy for eating. Most desserts have far more calories than that bread you just convinced yourself to avoid.

5. The Portion Habit

From time to time you will gain a pound or two. I like to weigh myself every morning to see if I need to go back to my "no snack" and "smaller portions" rules I used when losing weight. If I am a pound too heavy one morning, I revert to the "snack" and "portion" secrets I used in losing weight. It is much easier to maintain your weight a pound at a time than one day realizing you are five pounds over your goal weight. Don't ever forget the significance of portions.

6. No Calories from Beverages

Many individuals enjoy drinking Coca-Cola and other soft drinks—regular and diet. The weight-loss phase of the plan recommends that you drink no beverage that adds calories to your diet. Having said that, I will give you a personal example of when I do drink Coke with every calorie it has.

I travel overseas a lot, many times to third world countries. You do not drink water from the tap in third world countries because it is contaminated. You don't even use tap water to wash your toothbrush. When I travel to such places, a major intake of liquids is Coke. Let me tell you the reasoning.

I try to consume the least amount of food possible while traveling because so many times I have eaten foods that did not agree with my intestines. I have had bottled water that has not agreed with me (or at least I thought it was filtered clean and bottled). I read an article in the Nairobi, Kenya, newspaper, on the front page I might add, that reported a study they did in that city. Eight out of eleven bottled waters sold in restaurants there had regular impure tap water in them. They were sealed around the bottle cap, and they were delivered to your table sealed, but the water inside the bottle was from the tap. I also visited a Coca-Cola plant nearby and saw how they filtered all their water through several feet of sand, guaranteeing its safety. After reading the article in the newspaper, and seeing the plant, I began drinking Coke when I travel. Plus, from a medical standpoint, it has a similar number of electrolytes within it that a doctor uses to replace the electrolytes lost from diarrhea or dehydration. Coke is a good form of hydration when traveling.

One more personal Coca-Cola acknowledgment from a medical standpoint. In some of the more primitive locations I have visited as a physician, someone would be brought into the hospital severely dehydrated. These patients usually had been sick for a long period of time and had lost not only fluid but also essential electrolytes such as chloride, sodium, and potassium. Back home, I would start an IV in the large vein underneath their collarbone and give them replacement fluid that had plenty of these electrolytes plus sugar. However, at some bush hospitals, no such IV fluids are available. In most parts of the world you can get Coke in the middle of nowhere. Coke has similar electrolytes and sugar to the replacement IV I would give at home. I would get a Coke and have them begin sipping it, similar to an IV amount, until they became rehydrated with fluid plus electrolytes.

So, enough on Coke. Unless you're regularly traveling to a third world country, if you want to lose weight, don't take any calories from the liquids you drink. Don't add sugar to your coffee or tea. Even if you live in the South, don't order sweet tea.

7. Nothing Fried

Remember to think of fried foods as having about a third more calories than the same food not fried. But even more important than the calories, focus on the damaging saturated fat you are adding by frying whatever you are eating. Order baked potatoes rather than French fries. Order grilled rather than fried. You simply order or cook your meat grilled or sautéed in olive oil or canola oil if you want a change from simple grilling.

And don't forget to make certain you instruct whoever is taking your order to leave off the cream or cheese sauces that are added to so many grilled foods.

8. No Appetizer

No appetizer before your meal. There is no reason to go to a restaurant and order an appetizer and a salad, plus a main course, followed by dessert. Those days of ordering should be over as your new eating lifestyle takes control.

The *Moment* of Decision

As you develop your eating lifestyle you will realize that the foundation of your eating strategy is fruits, vegetables, and salads. For your rule of thumb on salads, remember that you can add almost as many calories as an entrée to your salad if you add cheese or regular dressing, both of which can also be very high in saturated fat.

You will still eat fish and chicken, but you will eat less of them. They will become more supplemental than primary items of your diet. They will become secondary to your meal rather than the primary food.

Last come soups. They can be a satisfying addition to your noon or evening meal. There is only one rule to go by—no cream-based or cheese soups.

These secrets and easy steps help you in the decisions you'll make as you work your Prescription for Life plan. The following is an encouragement from someone who took one of those decision moments and made something out of it.

Before dinner one evening, I was with someone I have known

for years. He had a 70 percent blockage in one of his heart arteries and was significantly overweight. He was asking me about the secret of losing weight, and I went over some of the ideas in the Prescription for Life plan.

At the end of our discussion, I mentioned that there was no doubt he could lose his excess weight. I explained that he could lose it all in just a moment of time. In "the twinkling of an eye" is the shortest time period I know of, and I told him that in the twinkling of an eye he could decide in his heart that he was going to reach his ideal weight. All he had to do was make such a decision and add commitment to it—and it would happen.

I will never forget the look on his face. His black hair was brushed back as if a hairstylist had just been working on it. His eyebrows were slightly raised, and his eyes opened wider than normal. He looked like someone had taken a flash picture and frozen it momentarily. He stared, without speaking a word. I had no idea what he was thinking or getting ready to say. His face finally broke into a half smile as he told me, "The next time you see me, I will be fifty pounds lighter." He concluded by telling me, "I really mean it."

When the waitress took our order that evening, I was amused at what he ordered—a tossed salad. He instructed the waitress to make sure it had no cheese and also to bring him a fat-free dressing.

Once we finished ordering, I took out a napkin and wrote on it his commitment to lose fifty pounds and slid it over to him. He smiled and initialed the statement and reminded me that it was going to happen. He is another one who made the decision in his mind, plus the commitment in his heart.

He is one who wanted no shame for staying overweight—and he did something about it.

How to Eat Once There

One morning, you will get up, look at the scale, and realize you are there. You have reached your ideal weight.

From that moment on, your eating strategy will change somewhat. The foods you will eat and the foods you will avoid do not change. That is the key difference in the Prescription for Life plan. You will have learned the foods that harm your arteries and will have developed many excellent eating habits that will never change again. There will be foods you used to crave, but now you will not care less whether you ever take another bite of them. You also will have developed a desire for certain foods that you never thought you would care for. You will continue eating very similarly to when you were losing your weight. You will go back to the weight-loss secrets and the easy steps for losing weight every time you realize you have gained a pound or two because your portions have been too large, or you have had too many snacks, or you haven't exercised as your routine calls for.

Once there, the two biggest changes you will make are reversing your weight-loss secrets concerning no snacks and small portions. The transition will be slow. You will add snacks if you really get hungry but not just because you want something to taste. And you will center your snacks on nuts and fruits. You will still eat smaller portions than you used to, but you will find yourself adjusting according to your daily weight.

Here is the good part. You won't change your regular eating strategy all that much from your weight-loss eating strategy. It will surprise you how food has become secondary in your thinking process. You won't live to eat certain foods you used to crave. You will have beaten your addiction and will be thankful you have taken control of your eating habits—for the remainder of your life.

Part 4

Exercise

Most people think of exercise as an activity that burns off calories, resulting in weight loss. That is true, but you need to grasp that there are so many more benefits from exercise. Once you know them, you will value your exercise time much more significantly. As a matter of fact, you will most likely not even place the calorie burn effect on the overall scale when weighing the benefits of exercise.

Most people also do not realize the dangers of *not exercising*. The life expectancy of those who are sedentary is comparable to those who smoke or have high blood pressure, yet few relate sitting on the couch to being that harmful. You are about to learn the huge effect exercise has on the most important organ of your body, your heart. You will understand why exercise extends your life expectancy significantly. You will learn on which cancers exercise has substantial protective effect. By the time you have read this part of the book, you will understand that calorie counts are significant but that you will enjoy many more benefits as you attack the aging factor head on—with *exercise*. Without exercise your chances of getting trim are slim.

17

The Most Unrecognized Way
to Combat Aging

"If you can't walk a quarter of a mile in five minutes, your chance of dying within three years is 30 percent greater than that of a faster walker." I was stunned when I read that introductory sentence in an article concerning the importance of exercise. And so I introduce you to perhaps the most significant segment of the Prescription for Life plan: exercise.

He was a little pudgy, but his slacks were neatly pressed and the buckle on his leather belt was real silver. I will never forget that day he showed me his exercise room. I'd been told how wealthy he was, about his house and cars and vacation spots. But until I actually saw his wood-paneled exercise room and his fancy mirrors and the pile of fresh towels stacked beside the water fountain, I couldn't imagine all the exercise equipment he had—anything money could buy. Every piece of exercise apparatus you would ever use was in place, and it all still looked new.

I asked him what his exercise routine was, and he said, "I don't really have a routine." "Really?" I questioned—a little surprised. The more we talked, the more I realized he exercised maybe once a month. Oh, he exercised a lot more when he initially bought the equipment; he was a good enough businessman to realize he needed to use the equipment because he had spent so much on it. But that was three years ago. I didn't say a word, but I kept thinking that even with his wealth, he couldn't buy health. It reminded me of Psalm 49:8–9: "No one can ever pay enough to live forever and never see the grave" (NLT). He couldn't buy a single extra day of life.

You can't buy health, but article after article in the medical literature substantiates that exercise has a powerful effect on the longevity and quality of your life. The *quality* of your life is so much more significant than the *length* of your life. All of us have seen individuals who are "alive," per se, but the quality of their lives is not optimal, and for many it is even terrible.

There is a difference between having a "physically active lifestyle" and a "personal exercise program." Being physically active rather than being completely sedentary is important, but having your own personal exercise program five to six days a week brings so many more rewards to your health. One of the best strategies for healthy years is to develop a lifestyle that includes exercise. Unless you develop an exercise program, your chances of getting to an ideal weight and eating properly are slim.

Don't Sabotage Your Exercise with Snacks

You burn around a hundred calories per mile whether you walk that mile or run it. Let's say you run three miles a day. That would be three hundred calories burned off. Even a light snack would counterbalance those three hundred calories very easily.

There is no way you are going to exercise enough to cover the extra calories you might be tempted to eat just in the form of snacks. Let me give you a few examples.

Assume you weigh 175 pounds and your exercise consists of walking. If you eat one slice of toast with jam on it, you will have to walk for 22 minutes to burn off the 125 calories. If you ran, it would be less: 13 minutes. One morning, you decide you would rather eat a 240-calorie donut instead of toast and jam. You will have to walk 42 minutes or run 18.

Then after dinner, you decide you want just one cup of ice cream. That's about 275 calories. That's another 48 minutes of walking or 20 minutes of running to burn those calories. An apple (70 calories): walk 12 minutes, run 5 minutes. And finally, one of your favorite candy bars. For the 270-calorie Snickers chocolate bar, you will have to walk the same as for the ice cream, 48 minutes, or run 20 minutes.

If there wasn't more to exercising than just burning off extra calories, it would never be worth exercising.

The Hidden Benefits of Exercise

A hidden benefit of exercise is that it convinces your mind you are serious about your overall healthy lifestyle. If you are putting thirty to sixty minutes a day, five to six days per week, into your exercise routine, you are very serious about your overall lifestyle decision. Dedication to exercise convinces your mind that you intend to stay at an ideal weight, that you are serious about what you are going to eat and what you are not going to eat. It's a great reinforcement.

Exercise may not be something you look forward to every day. Sometimes it can be a chore to go to the gym, or to get on your treadmill, or to go to a park or track so you can run. But the big reward comes when you feel so much better afterward.

I will never forget when Jack LaLanne celebrated his ninetieth birthday. He had been an exercise guru back before many people were intentionally exercising. I can still picture him when he was interviewed on television. Three people were talking about all he had done to get Americans into exercise programs over the years.

When he walked out on the stage, he held up his arms and flexed his biceps for all to see. He looked to be about seventy, not ninety. After he sat down, the interviewer asked him how old he was. He smiled as he said, "None of your business." He was then asked what exercises he did on a near daily basis, and he went into detail about his core muscles and weight lifting and what he did to get his heart rate up to a certain level. One of the interviewers stated that it was so great seeing someone his age who enjoyed his daily exercise routine. His response was priceless.

"Enjoy it?" He leaned forward in his seat like he was about ready to reach out and hit her. "I don't enjoy it one minute. I hate exercise. I do not like getting up and going to the gym to work out. I hate it." He paused and smiled. "But I do like the great feeling I get when I'm through."

To me, that answer says it all. Exercise may not be something you like doing, but you are committed to doing it. It is like going to work. You may not want to go in on a particular morning, but you do it. And you like it when you receive your paycheck. Same way with exercise; commit to it and stick with it. You will indeed enjoy a great reward for doing it. Plus, it's a great paycheck.

The medical literature gives conclusive evidence that there is a direct relationship between one's weight and whether they exercise. The consensus is that the more one is physically active, the less body weight they have. Physically active people weigh less than people who are not active. Many studies show that if you use exercise as part of your weight-loss program and then quit the exercise, your weight will go back up.

I remind you of a study mentioned earlier. Remember the Brown University study in which one group of overweight women dieted only and the other group dieted *and* exercised? The group that dieted and exercised lost almost twice the weight in comparison to the ones who dieted without exercising. If you don't remember any other report, keep this one in the forefront of your mind when you think about losing weight.

Developing the Right Program for You

Your exercise program will be of your own design because everyone is different physically and may choose different exercise routines. The Prescription for Life plan is a general one that anyone can plug in to. If you are obese or sedentary, it may be all you can do to begin walking for thirty minutes a day. It doesn't matter so much *where* you start as *that* you start. So start walking.

You may be able to lift only a two-pound weight over your head three times before your muscles give out. You may have trouble getting your leg over the seat of a stationary bicycle, and once on, you may be out of breath in three minutes. Start where your body will let you. And your goal will be to eat the right foods and exercise in conjunction with each other to get the weight off. The day will come when you will be halfway to your ideal weight, on a treadmill at a brisk walk, checking your heart rate to get it above the 80th percentile of the maximum rate, and you will look in the mirror—and smile.

Weight loss. Exercise.
Exercise. Weight loss.

You may not be overweight one ounce, but if you're not exercising you are missing out on one of the greatest health benefits you can have. Not exercising costs you more than you would ever imagine. The great majority of people have no idea the passive damage you bring on your body by not being active. Inactivity is one of the key causes of physiological aging.

18

The Sedentary Life of a Couch Potato

Exercise is a key component to helping your body remain as young physiologically as possible. Whether you're extremely active or you do no exercise at all, you need to read this section to understand the connection between exercise and your health.

The Prescription for Life program begins with a plan that even a couch potato can start. It is that simple. And whether your activity level is anywhere from minimum to running eight-minute miles every day, you will be able to plug in to the plan at whatever stage you are in.

Numerous reports in the medical literature show that being sedentary is as much of a risk factor for disease in your heart or brain as is smoking or having high blood pressure. If you know how bad smoking is to your physical condition and realize what high blood pressure does to your arteries, you know why you don't want to have a lifestyle that can cause similar problems.

Sedentary. Look it up in the dictionary. It's an adjective that describes a person who does a lot of sitting and correspondingly little exercise.

These same studies on exercise show that two-thirds of Americans are not active on a regular basis and over half of Americans are completely sedentary.

The Sedentary Lifestyle Is as Dangerous as Smoking

Most everyone realizes that smoking and high blood pressure are two of the greatest risk factors that compound any effect LDL Cholesterol has on your arteries. In all my years of practice, I found that smoking is the single most detrimental activity to the human body. I operated on lung cancer patients and saw how smoking affected them, inside and out. If the cancer is caught early enough, it can be cured. If it has already spread through the lymph nodes and throughout the body, your time is limited. Most of my lung cancer patients quit smoking after their operation. But even after an operation, some continued smoking because they could not beat their addiction. A sedentary lifestyle can be similar to such an addiction.

Reports state that being inactive affects your body similarly to smoking. In other words, the potential consequences of both are similar. Smoking causes emphysema, which makes the simple act of breathing extremely difficult. You can't get fresh air in and you can't get stale air out. Your chest expands as much as it can, trying to pull more air in—but to no avail. You end up taking short, shallow breaths and have to breathe twice as rapidly to move what little air you can. Smoking causes cancer. Smoking plays a part in causing high blood pressure.

Inactivity can cause health problems that are different from smoking but are equally as damaging to your body. Inactivity can lead to death—or even worse. It can leave you with so many ailments that it almost becomes not worth fighting to live.

One needs to realize that the overall health of a sedentary person is no better than that of someone who smokes. You are thinking that being sedentary doesn't cause you to have difficulty breathing. And it doesn't the same way cigarette smoking does. But if you medically study sedentary patients, you will find health problem numbers similar to those of smokers. The couch potato usually gets overweight, frequently develops diabetes and high blood pressure, and ends up with a heart attack or stroke. There are so many secondary diseases associated with being sedentary that the numbers closely resemble those seen by people who smoke.

Acknowledge what game you are playing with your body when you remain sedentary. The bottom line damage to your overall health is similar to the damage caused by smoking.

The Sedentary Lifestyle Is as Risky as High Blood Pressure

Physiologically, it is as bad to be sedentary as it is to have high blood pressure. Everyone realizes the dangers of high blood pressure and will take whatever medication to get it down as close to the normal range as possible. Patients realize that if it goes untreated, it can become fatal. Most people understand that high blood pressure is a common cause of strokes. High blood pressure compounds the problem of LDL in your arteries. Any patient I ever knew who smoked and also had high blood pressure would take medication for their blood pressure, even if they didn't quit smoking.

Everyone opts to do something about their high blood pressure, but not everyone opts to do something about their sedentary lifestyle. And such a lifestyle is equally as bad. Take your medicine—exercise. It's as simple as doing something to increase your activity.

The Framingham Heart Study shows that something as simple as brisk walking for thirty minutes daily can increase your life expectancy by years. Brisk walking doesn't seem like much exercise compared to running a marathon. But when you've made thirty minutes of brisk walking a day your goal, you've done so much more than extend your life expectancy. Such individuals also set as their goals to eat the right foods and to work toward an ideal weight. Set your sights on briskly walking thirty minutes a day, then as time goes by, mix in a slow jog, and as time goes on, continue to increase your pace on the treadmill.

A nine-year study compared people who were sedentary with those who were moderately fit. Everyone knows that people who smoke, have high cholesterol, or have high blood pressure have a higher premature death rate than those who don't. But look at this: even if someone does smoke or has elevated cholesterol or high blood pressure but is actively fit, their premature death rate is better than a sedentary person's who also smokes, has elevated blood pressure, or has elevated cholesterol. That says a lot about the significance of exercise, even if you aren't taking proper care of your health otherwise.

You can't imagine how significant not exercising is. The more active you become, the better the arteries to your heart and brain are going to be and the younger you are going to be physiologically.

Most people, at one time or another, have worked on changing their diets to lose weight. But not enough have thought of exercise as an important factor in losing weight and improving health.

Putting both strategies together makes a huge impact. Your diet is paramount in decreasing your LDL Cholesterol—and exercise is tops in increasing your HDL Cholesterol.

19

Why Exercise Is So Good for You

You add years to your life expectancy by exercising. Now you are going to find out *why* that is true. Here are three factors to keep in mind:

1. To improve your health and longevity, decrease your lethal LDL Cholesterol and increase your healthy HDL Cholesterol.
2. The primary factor in keeping your LDL down is to avoid certain bad foods.
3. The primary factor in elevating your HDL is exercise.

Exercise raises your HDL, and the more vigorous, the better. I know a friend who decided to begin jogging and set three miles as his goal. He told me that on the first day he made it to his neighbor's mailbox. The second day he ran twice as far and soon was able to run a whole block. (By the way, he did walk for a total of three miles each of those days.) He did get to the point where he was running three miles a day at a nice clip. Get off the couch and begin, no matter how long it takes to get to your neighbor's mailbox. Set aside thirty minutes, and start being active in some way. Look at how exercise is such a protective factor for your arteries.

The Effect of Exercise on HDL Cholesterol

A study published in the *New England Journal of Medicine* gives a good summary concerning the relationship between exercise *intensity* and cholesterol. Some of the facts show the significance researchers placed on which type of exercise was performed. There were three exercise groups.

Their most active group was labeled "high-amount-high-intensity exercise." This group was equivalent to jogging approximately 20 miles a week at 65 to 80 percent peak oxygen consumption (pretty heavy exercise).

The second group was labeled "low-amount-high-intensity exercise," and that was the equivalent to jogging approximately 12 miles a week at 65 to 80 percent peak oxygen consumption.

And the third group was labeled "low-amount-moderate-intensity exercise," with the equivalent of walking approximately 12 miles a week at 40 to 55 percent peak oxygen consumption.

All in all, you can see that there is a significant difference in the amount of exercise each group did: (1) jogging 20 miles, fast pace; (2) jogging 12 miles, fast pace; and (3) walking 12 miles.

This study concluded that exercise definitely has a beneficial effect on cholesterol numbers. And the greater amount the exercise, the greater effect there is on the HDL/Total Cholesterol ratio score.

What caught my attention was that the LDL Cholesterol numbers came down but not nearly as significantly as the HDL Cholesterol numbers went up. The report showed a clear beneficial effect on the HDL Cholesterol, especially in the high-amount-high-intensity group: the greater the exercise, the greater the effect on raising their HDL, which affected the ratio of HDL to LDL significantly.

Other studies show as much as a 4 to 6 percent rise in HDL even with light exercise, such as stroller walkers and brisk walkers.

Your HDL level is profoundly related to protecting the blockage and inflammatory process in your arteries. This is substantiated by statements found in the *Third Report of the National Cholesterol Education Program Expert Panel on Detection, Evaluation, and Treatment of High Blood Cholesterol in Adults.* This is one of the most comprehensive studies on cholesterol in medical literature. First, researchers show strong evidence that low levels of HDL Cholesterol are associated with an increase in deaths related to coronary heart disease. They also point out the other side of the coin by stating that high HDL Cholesterol levels result in a reduced risk. This emphasizes that the health of your arteries is directly related to your HDL level.

They also stressed that physical inactivity has a similar artery disease risk as do smoking and diabetes.

Another study reported in the *Archives of Internal Medicine* reviewed articles from multiple medical journals to evaluate the effect of exercise on HDL and what protection that has on arteries. This review shows that with exercise, the HDL Cholesterol number is raised a little over two and a half points. Researchers then correlated this finding with another study, which had studied how beneficial it is to raise HDL even a single point. That correlation showed that for every point elevation of HDL Cholesterol, there is a 2 to 3 percent less chance of developing coronary heart disease of the arteries. The term they used in stating that exercise increases one's HDL Cholesterol was "highly significant."

Their recommended minimal exercise period was 120 minutes of weekly exercise—equal to thirty minutes a day, four days a week. But they pointed out that more is even better.

To put into perspective how much you could expect your HDL to increase as you exercise more, they found that for every ten minutes above that 120-minute minimum weekly exercise, you can expect nearly a one and a half point net increase in your HDL number. That means if you exercise thirty minutes a day for six days a week, you can raise your HDL in the neighborhood of ten points. Remember also that you get bonus points if you lose weight at the same time you are exercising. Such an increase has a significant effect on your HDL/Total Cholesterol ratio.

This all becomes more noteworthy when you fit it into your Prescription for Life plan. Not only are you improving your arteries by raising your HDL Cholesterol, but you are also getting added protection by combining exercise with weight loss. Add to that the improvement you get by avoiding the foods that raise the lethal LDL Cholesterol particles. Then you begin to realize that disease of the arteries of the heart and brain can be avoided and how each lifestyle change compounds the protective action on your health.

As the infomercials say, "But wait, there's more!" Exercise does even more than just increase your HDL Cholesterol.

Exercise and Cardiac Output

Your heart is the most important organ in your body, and how much you exercise plays a major role in its efficiency. Put your thinking cap on for this one. You are going to learn the great benefit exercise has on your heart, as a pump. Your heart pumps approximately 104,000 times a day, 38 million times a year, and is the primary organ responsible for furnishing nutrition and oxygen for your body.

I didn't know these precise numbers at the time, but the thought of how many times my heart had to beat precisely to keep the proper amount of blood pumping throughout my body kept entering my mind whenever I would pass a pumping station along the Alaska Pipeline route. You may remember seeing the ice road truckers on television, the people who haul supplies in Alaska above the Arctic Circle to Prudhoe Bay. Well, some friends and I rode our motorcycles up that Haul Road one summer, all the way up to Prudhoe Bay, where the pipeline begins.

The pipeline is eight hundred miles long, carrying oil from the Alaska oil fields down to Valdez. As I rode along, I began thinking of the similarity of those pipelines to the arteries of our bodies and how the oil pumping stations along the way operate similarly to the pumping action of our hearts. I realized that the most significant parts of that entire project were the pumping stations that are placed approximately twenty miles apart. Those pumps make the entire system work. They are positioned throughout the length of the pipeline to adjust the pressure and pump the oil along the line.

If a pump becomes weak or inefficient, the entire system will shut down. A plugged pump is the equivalent of a heart attack. Whenever any pump accidently shuts down, all focus centers on getting it repaired and back to work. And in an area where the record temperature reaches minus 72 degrees, such repairs could take days and days. So they do everything possible to keep the efficiency at peak. They practice prevention of pump shut down better than most people protect their hearts. They do whatever is needed to ensure that each pump stays in premier shape. Their primary goal is to not let a pump shut down.

Apply this concept to your heart. If you don't take proper care of your heart pump, your project will also shut down. However, there is a huge difference between the pipeline pumping stations and your heart. They can spend two days battling the cold and finally get a pump running again, whereas if your pump stops, you die.

So listen up and see how exercise makes your heart pump more efficiently. A conglomerate of reports shows that exercise will do two things to your heart muscle. First, your heart will pump more blood with fewer contraction beats because it will become stronger with exercise. And second, it will pump blood more efficiently because your heart muscle isn't going to need as much oxygen as the inefficient heart muscle of someone who is sedentary. Basically, the heart muscle of someone who exercises properly is so strong that it requires less oxygen to make it beat each time. It's like an engine in an automobile that is so efficient it can get thirty miles per gallon of gas versus a less efficient engine that gets only twenty.

With those two factors in mind, let's see what the studies show concerning the result of exercise on the efficiency of the heart.

First, researchers have found that exercise increases the amount of blood ejected by the heart per minute. This is called your *cardiac output*. Of course, if your heart is stronger, it can pump a greater amount of blood per minute.

Stay with me. It gets a little involved, but I want you to understand that the stronger your heart muscle is, the less oxygen your heart muscle requires. If you take your heart rate and multiply that number by the top number of your blood pressure, you get what is called the *index of oxygen demand*. That number gives you an indication of how much oxygen is required by that heart muscle before it runs out of oxygen and quits working. In essence, the exercised, stronger heart muscle requires less oxygen to carry on its work than the weaker, sedentary heartmuscle.

The stronger heart muscle, which is developed from exercise, requires less oxygen to pump an equal amount of blood than a weaker heart muscle. Reports show that a heart with a strong muscle needs only about half of the oxygen required by one not made strong by exercise.

The most significant medical advice in this regard is don't chance waiting for symptoms before doing something about protecting your heart.

The second most significant medical advice is if symptoms do occur and you are told you have had a light attack, or you have to have a stent placed, or even a bypass operation, there are immediate measures you must take to protect your future.

Whether you have had very little blockage or more severe obstruction, once the event is over, exercise has a most significant positive effect on the muscle of your heart.

A study of almost five thousand patients evaluated the benefit of exercise *after* a cardiac event. It was reported in the medical journal *Circulation*. The overall result was that cardiac rehabilitation with exercise resulted in approximately a 20 percent reduction in total mortality and a 26 percent reduction in cardiac mortality. If you, or someone you know, have experienced a cardiac event, take that statement as a flashing, neon warning sign. Obviously, reduction in mortality means reduction in dying.

But the same study showed a difference in the chance of having another heart attack, even if the people studied didn't die from it. It showed that cardiac rehabilitation with exercise resulted in approximately a 27 percent reduction in having another cardiac event compared to rehabilitation that did not include exercise. Exercise is one of those "have-to" factors if you have had a heart event. If you know someone who has had a stent or heart attack, remind them of this. They may even thank you for the information.

Also interesting is that, in the exercise group of the study, there were not only fewer recurring cardiac events but also fewer times those patients had to be rehospitalized. The basis for this is that exercise reduced the number of patients who developed angina, which required them to be hospitalized. Angina is what happens if an artery in the heart is partially blocked but not enough to cause the muscle to die. It is almost to that point but not quite there just yet. The muscle not getting enough oxygen begins to cause pain, but enough blood gets through to not shut the muscle down completely. The resulting angina pain creates a transient chest pain. Some describe heaviness or a discomfort in their chest, a burning sensation or a squeezing of their chest. Angina blockage is the lightest blockage and is usually a precursor to a full-blown heart attack waiting to happen. The report showed that exercise reduces the number of these angina attacks, thus, fewer hospitalizations.

Another extremely significant finding is that those same patients who exercised *plus* ate properly had even fewer subsequent stent placements and bypass operations. In other words, the report stressed the significance of the importance of overall lifestyle changes of both exercising and eating properly.

The bottom line of all these studies is that people who change their lifestyle after a heart attack or stent placement to include regular exercise have improved rates of survival. If you, or anyone you know, have had heart artery problems, get with a physician and get into a rehab program that includes exercise. And if you haven't had symptoms of blockage of your arteries, get to work on *preventing* it ever getting to that point. Take these studies to heart—literally.

20

The Exercise Plan
Everyone Can Follow

The following exercise plan is going to work for you, whether you are a couch potato or already exercise every day. The plan consists of two types of exercise. One will be exercising your heart, called *aerobic* exercise. The other will be muscular fitness, or *anaerobic* exercise. You will be doing both, but aerobic is the most important because that is the one that keeps your pump working at its peak. Everyone can fit into a particular phase of the plan.

Heed the warnings about being inactive. Inactivity, the couch potato syndrome, is an independent risk factor for heart disease. Inactivity is not a zero on the health scale; it is a minus.

Exercise strengthens your heart.

It lowers your heart rate.

It lowers your blood pressure.

It lowers the oxygen demand of your heart muscle.

Do it.

Aerobic Exercise

Aerobic exercise not only strengthens your heart muscle but also helps you lose weight, lower your blood pressure, and decrease your risk of heart attack, stroke, diabetes, and even some cancers.

Aerobic exercise is so important because it keeps your most physically important organ going at top efficiency. The stronger the pump, the easier it is to get blood flowing throughout your body. Remember my telling you about anatomy class that first week in medical school? Why were the muscles of some heart walls only a few millimeters thick while others were ten to twenty times thicker? That was back in medical school, but when I started my surgical rotations through cardiac surgery, I began understanding what made the difference. The heart muscle is just like any other muscle. If it is forced to exercise at least at a minimum on most days, the muscle grows thicker.

Strengthening your heart muscle is similar to strengthening your biceps. The more you exercise it, the thicker and stronger the heart muscle gets. If you put a work force on the muscle, it responds by getting stronger. The more the work force you place on your heart, the more times it will beat per minute during that work force. When you die, you want the pathologist to look at your heart and remark how thick and strong that muscle looks.

Jogging is one of the best ways to strengthen your heart because it keeps your heart at an elevated sustained heart rate for a specific period of time. You will agree with this statement after we review the following report written in the journal *Archives of Internal Medicine*.

The study, which began in 1976, involved twenty thousand men and women. Their ages ranged from twenty to ninety-three. The study compared a subgroup of joggers to a subgroup of non-joggers. What differences they found between the two groups is significant. The joggers were asked about their jogging intensity and speed and the time they spent jogging each week. The investigators based their results on the ones who jogged between one hour and two and a half hours a week. (That's thirty minutes a day, two to five days a week.) The intensity of this jogging group was not that great, but what was impressive was how much better off they were than the group that did not jog at all.

There was a significant increase in life expectancy for the group that jogged. The study showed that the risk of death was reduced by 44 percent in the jogging group. That number jumped out at me, but the next point is what really got my attention. *The data showed that jogging was linked with an added 6.2 years to the life expectancies for men and 5.6 years to the life expectancies for women.*

This study clearly shows the importance of exercise. But the real question is, *Why* does jogging actually extend your life? The answer is found in many studies that explain that jogging raises HDL, which in turn protects your arteries.

Not only does it extend your life by giving you more HDL police car molecules to carry off the LDL splinters stuck in your arteries, but also helps extend your life by preventing obesity and increasing bone density, as well as by improving psychological function and lowering your triglycerides.

The most significant reason exercise such as jogging extends your life is that it strengthens your heart muscle. The reasoning goes like this: the best exercise you can do to strengthen your heart is to sustain a significantly high heart rate for a thirty-minute interval. Multiple trials show that maximum strength of your heart muscle is obtained by keeping the heart rate above the eightieth percentile of your maximum rate during that interval.

Most of the reports are based on individuals who run five or six days per week. It is easy to figure the eightieth percentile number of your maximum heart rate. This is a rule of thumb way to do it, but it is very workable.

Take the number 220, subtract your age, and that will give what your maximum heart rate should be. That doesn't mean your heart will stop if you go one beat over, but it is a good number to work with. Then, take 80 percent of that maximum heart rate number to obtain the number you should aim to sustain during your exercise period.

After reading several articles concerning sustaining my heart rate above the eightieth percentile, I bought the first of several pulse counting wristwatches I have owned over the years. I began a jogging routine of running three miles and have persisted in that routine ever since. Your *resting heart rate* is the bottom-line test of how strong your heart muscle is. It wasn't long before my resting heart rate was in the 40 to 44 range. After years of exercising above my eightieth percentile, I'm dying to know how thick my heart muscle is but not necessarily willing to let some medical school anatomy professor find out for me anytime soon.

Set thirty minutes a day as your aerobic exercise period, whether you are walking or jogging. If you haven't jogged before, begin with a brisk walk for thirty minutes a day. No matter where you are on the fitness continuum, the important word is *begin*. Your walk can be done on a track or a treadmill or a path, then slowly increase your pace over several weeks. Then jog intermittently for several-minute intervals during your brisk thirty-minute walk and you will eventually end up with the full half hour—jogging or running. All the while, you are keeping your heart rate above your eightieth percentile, and your heart is getting stronger and stronger.

Any way you look at it, exercise is a great investment—with a payoff of adding 6.2 years to the life expectancies of men and 5.6 years to the life expectancies of women.

There is a good self-test to determine if you are exercising enough to get your heart muscle working at peak performance. You can do it after you finish your brisk walk or fast jog, or whatever you are doing that gets your heart rate above the eightieth percentile range. After finishing your thirty minutes, count your pulse at the end of one minute and again at the end of two minutes. As your heart muscle gets toward optimum strength, your pulse rate will drop more and more dramatically just after completing your exercise. You will know your heart muscle is at its peak performance when you find that your rate drops twenty-five beats by the end of the first minute after completing your aerobic exercise and drops an additional fifteen beats by the end of your second minute.

Again, these are round numbers, but they will give you a great indication as to how well you are doing with the aerobic portion of your exercise routine. When you get your heart muscle to the strongest point, you will consistently hit the twenty-five-beat decrease after the first minute and the fifteen-beat decrease at the end of two minutes after completing your jog or run.

Aerobic Exercise Plan

The plan is based on thirty minutes a day, six days a week. It has been shown that cardiac strengthening exercise for more than thirty minutes does not significantly further improve the strength of your heart. You can run longer, but don't think of it as significantly helping your heart more than if you ran for only thirty minutes.

Let's begin with a plan to get you moving if exercise is new for you. If you cannot jog yet, simply begin with a thirty-minute walk every day at a steady pace for a one-week period. The following week, move to a faster walk, and eventually to a brisk walk. On a treadmill, a brisk walk is three to four miles per hour. *Committing to a thirty-minute walk may be the most significant decision you ever make.* You will have "begun." The goal will be more vigorous activity, but don't let that discourage you. Do what you can do and keep working to improve. Your initial goal is being able to jog for two minutes. Then you move into the regular plan below.

Not long ago I was sitting in a lounge chair on the beach watching an obese woman in her midthirties walking approximately fifty yards and then running as hard as she could for about fifteen strides. She repeated this time and again all the way down the beach. I wanted to jump out of my chair and go congratulate her on her exercise program. It may have been her first day; I don't know. But she was doing something about getting in better health.

So don't feel discouraged when we discuss more vigorous exercise. It doesn't matter where you are on the exercise continuum; just commit to starting a thirty-minute program. Remember, there is much more to it than just how vigorous your exercise is. Your thirty minutes of exercise sends a huge message to your brain about your commitment to eating the proper foods and getting to your ideal weight, no matter how fast you are moving. The main thing is to commit to your own thirty-minute exercise program and get started with it.

Even if you already exercise regularly, the following plan is also for you. You can fit yourself into this scheme no matter what your exercise status happens to presently be. However, if you are a couch potato, you must begin with a commitment to

Thirty-Minute Walk/Jog

Week	Day 1	Day 2	Day 3	Day 4	Day 5	Day 6	Day 7
1	2 min jog 28 min brisk walk	2 min jog 28 min brisk walk	2 min jog 28 min brisk walk	3 min jog 27 min brisk walk	3 min jog 27 min brisk walk	3 min jog 27 min brisk walk	rest
2	4 min jog 26 min brisk walk	4 min jog 26 min brisk walk	4 min jog 26 min brisk walk	5 min jog 25 min brisk walk	5 min jog 25 min brisk walk	5 min jog 25 min brisk walk	rest
3	6 min jog 24 min brisk walk	6 min jog 24 min brisk walk	6 min jog 24 min brisk walk	7 min jog 23 min brisk walk	7 min jog 23 min brisk walk	7 min job 23 min brisk walk	rest
4	8 min jog 22 min brisk walk	8 min jog 22 min brisk walk	8 min jog 22 min brisk walk	9 min jog 21 min brisk walk	9 min jog 21 min brisk walk	9 min jog 21 min brisk walk	rest
5	10 min jog 20 min brisk walk	10 min jog 20 min brisk walk	10 min jog 20 min brisk walk	12 min jog 18 min brisk walk	12 min jog 18 min brisk walk	12 min jog 18 min brisk walk	rest
6	14 min jog 16 min brisk walk	14 min jog 16 min brisk walk	14 min jog 16 min brisk walk	16 min jog 14 min brisk walk	16 min jog 14 min brisk walk	16 min jog 14 min brisk walk	rest
7	18 min jog 12 min brisk walk	18 min jog 12 min brisk walk	18 min jog 12 min brisk walk	20 min jog 10 min brisk walk	20 min jog 10 min brisk walk	20 min jog 10 min brisk walk	rest
8	22 min jog 8 min brisk walk	22 min jog 8 min brisk walk	22 min jog 8 min brisk walk	24 min jog 6 min brisk walk	24 min jog 6 min brisk walk	24 min jog 6 min brisk walk	rest
9	26 min jog 4 min brisk walk	26 min jog 4 min brisk walk	26 min jog 4 min brisk walk	28 min jog 2 min brisk walk	28 min jog 2 min brisk walk	28 min jog 2 min brisk walk	rest
10	30 min jog	30 min jog	30 min jog	30 min jog	30 min jog	30 min jog	rest

begin walking for thirty minutes and then advance to a brisk walk. The chart on page 234 is the next step after you have conquered the thirty minutes of brisk walking. It begins with a two-minute jog followed by twenty-eight minutes of brisk walking. See where you fit and get started.

Again, the plan takes thirty minutes a day, six days a week. Warm up and stretch before you jog and again after you walk or jog. By the way, I know there are reports that you don't need to stretch before you run, but the same people still say you should walk five minutes before taking off running. I haven't found much comment in the leading medical journals about all this, so I still like to get my muscles and ligaments stretched out completely before putting them to work.

Your jog pace is up to you and your ability. If you are already active, your plan is simply to enter the above scheme at your present exercise level. If you aren't yet jogging for thirty minutes, count the minutes you can jog and fit that time into the above plan. As an example, if you are able to run ten minutes without stopping, you fit into the week five plan. Then progress from there as the plan moves on to week six.

For those who complete week ten, when you are jogging for thirty minutes, plus for those who already can jog for thirty minutes, the second stage of the plan takes over. At that point, you change from thinking time to thinking distance, going from minutes to miles. You go from having a goal of thirty minutes to a goal of three miles. After being able to jog thirty consecutive minutes, you begin focusing on increasing your jogging pace. Use three miles as the limit for distance. If you can run three miles in less than thirty minutes, you can stop at the three-mile point, even if the time is less than thirty minutes.

Set your own personal goals. But above all else, get off the couch and get started.

Heart Strength Indicator

The best indicator of cardiac strength is your resting heart rate. Lie down for at least ten minutes and then take your pulse to find your resting heart rate. The stronger your heart muscle, the lower your resting heart rate will be. A normal resting heart rate is usually stated as 72, but a strong muscle doesn't have to contract as often to pump the same volume of blood as a weaker muscle, thus a slower pulse beat per minute. The stronger your muscle, the lower your resting heart rate is. If your heart is near perfect strength condition, your rate will be in the 40 beats per minute range.

A strong heart doesn't have to contract as many times to pump the same amount of blood throughout the body as a weaker heart. Now think of that same principle all night long, while your body is at rest. The normal sequence is for the heart muscle to contract and then get to rest after each contraction. If the normal heart rate is 72 times a minute to pump a certain amount of blood through your body, it is getting to rest only the amount of time between each of those 72 beats. An exercised heart muscle can pump the same amount of blood, contracting only 40 times a minute, as a nonexercised heart that pumps 72 times a minute. That leaves a longer time interval between each beat for the exercised heart to rest. It is getting to rest almost twice as long beating 40 times a minute as a normal heart beating 72 times a minute.

Even I could run a marathon if I got to stop and rest numerous times throughout the race and still finish with the same time as everyone else running.

Your resting heart rate is an excellent way to know whether you are exercising the amount you need to get your HDL to the highest level. Whether you swim, cycle, or jog—outside or on a treadmill—increase your heart rate by exercising to strengthen your cardiac output ability. Test that strength by counting your resting heart rate.

Anaerobic Exercise

The anaerobic part of your exercise plan can be varied enough to fit your personal taste. If you go to a gym, you have numerous machines to choose from. If you exercise at home, you can get some basic light weights and a weight bench. A wraparound ankle belt to use for leg extension exercise is also good to have. You can use rubber resistance bands or weights that wrap around your ankles with Velcro.

As you age, unless you do something about it, time will take a toll on the quality of your muscles. If you do not do the strength training of anaerobic exercise, your muscles will become weaker. That will lead to more difficulty in handling everyday tasks, more chance of falling and of bone fractures, and you will even become more fatigued doing your normal everyday activities. You will become older and older. Most people get less active as they become older, but from a physical standpoint, you don't have to.

About 70 percent of the strength you lose is due to a decline in physical activity. You can avoid this by doing anaerobic exercises to keep your muscles strong. Don't fall into the trap most people do as they get older, the trap of becoming more sedentary. Begin your anaerobic exercise program to keep your muscles toned and strong. You will walk better, have better posture, and feel better about yourself. Your muscles are responsible for every move you make. The stronger the muscles, the easier to live the life you want to enjoy.

This anaerobic plan focuses on strength training. You have seen pictures of younger individuals with huge bicep muscles, their chests and necks looking like an engine coming toward you, and their abs looking like well-built, firmly padded ladders. They get that way with anaerobic exercise. Such individuals are strengthening each muscle repetitively, until each muscle fiber enlarges. They are not making any new muscles. They are just developing the individual muscle fibers that are already present, to the fullest extent.

Even though the cardio part of the exercise program should receive at least 80 percent of your attention, the anaerobic program should not be taken lightly. It is important for balance, for movement, for coordination, and for overall agility. It is one of the best ways to slow the decline of muscle mass that occurs as you get older. It is best to start an anaerobic exercise program as early as possible, but it is never too late to begin.

Not only does exercise improve your muscles, but it is also the number one way you can stimulate bone density. Exercise stresses your muscles, but it also places stress on your bones. That is extremely important because it helps to increase bone density and reduce the risk of osteoporosis. If you are on a calcium supplement of some type, ask your doctor if you need to continue it if you have an exercise program.

There are many programs for each set of muscles, and I will leave the specifics up to you as to what you want to incorporate into your strategy for exercise. But your overall aim is to complete one set of exercises for each of your major muscle groups. There are many ways to do this, but work on something you can do that includes your shoulders, chest, back, arms, abdomen, and legs. Keep it simple and write down a routine.

Legs

Starting with the lower body, one of the most significant exercises to protect your knees is leg extension exercise. If you go to a gym, there are specific machines where you can slide the front of your ankles behind a padded bar and then extend the bar by straightening out your legs. This stresses the quadriceps muscles, which are the large group of muscles on the front of your thighs. The reason it is so important to exercise these is that they end in tendons that strap around each side of your knee. Think of it as an exterior steel cage surrounding your knee, protecting those smaller, finer ligaments located within your knee joint. It is the inner ligaments that become torn so easily and cause so much difficulty.

If you don't go to a gym, you can buy ankle weights, which you wrap around your ankle. Sitting in a chair, lift and fully flex your knee and grasp your leg behind and just above your knee. Then repeatedly extend your knee from that position.

Arms, Shoulders, Lateral Chest, Back

These exercises can be performed with weight lifting machines or with free weights. You can flex your biceps with a repetition of weights in each hand. The same weights can be used laterally for chest muscle strength and directly overhead for shoulder strengthening exercises. Push-ups are another good exercise to add to your overall routine.

Here is one rule of thumb to keep in mind with weight lifting: if you are using free weights, select a weight—or a resistance level if you are using a machine—that feels heavy enough so that by about the twelfth to fifteenth repetition you are barely able to finish it. Some may be able to begin with only 2 or 3 pounds. That's fine, just continue to progress and you will eventually find a comfortable weight you can do on a regular basis. As your muscles strengthen with continued exercise, it will surprise you how you progress.

Core Muscles

Most people focus on their arms, shoulders, chest, and legs. But you use the core muscles of your body to coordinate movement every time you take a step or reach up to get a glass out of a cabinet. Your core muscles in the midsection of your body make all kinds of adjustments to support your body as it moves. They are the foundation all these movements are built upon.

Again, if you go to a gym, you can use their machines designed specifically for this. The basic one is where you sit with your back to the weight machine and pull two straps over your shoulders and bend forward, pulling a certain amount of weight against your abdominal muscles.

At home, many do crunches, where you lie on your back and raise your shoulders off the floor and repeatedly tighten your abdominal muscles. A variation of that is to lie on the floor with your shoulders and feet both raised so you are resting solely on your buttocks. This is followed by repeatedly pulling your knees toward your chest as you extend your arms forward, much like a rowing motion.

Back Paraspinal Muscles

So many people complain of difficulty with their backs. Yet in exercise books you will find very little written about how to strengthen the muscles of your back. And to top that off, many of the exercises focus on stretching the back muscles by leaning forward. That stretches the back muscles but doesn't flex them. The muscles that hold your back erect are located on each side of your spine. And, of course, they are located on the back side of the spine. If you bend forward, you are stretching these muscles. You are not flexing them except when you straighten up your back after bending forward. To add strength to these muscles, they need to be flexed. The following is the best exercise I have found to strengthen your back.

I learned it in the Air Force. After completing surgery training, I served for two years at the Air Force Academy Hospital in Colorado. While I was there, they allowed officers to participate in the cadets' free-fall parachute jump school once a year. You had to be able to run three miles at a seven-minute-a-mile pace to be accepted, so you had to be in excellent physical condition to take the course. It was the only place in the United States where the very first jump was a solo, free-fall jump, with a ten-second delay before opening your chute.

The jump school class lasted several weeks. You did simulated jumps from towers, learned the proper techniques of how to reach for your pull line to deploy the chute, and learned from what seemed like at least a thousand death-defying instructions. The only thing we didn't have to learn was how to pack our chute, because they had a trusted expert who did that for us. (It was my guess that they were afraid we wouldn't do it properly and the chute wouldn't open.)

One of the most significant aspects of the jump was the posture for your free fall. Your back had to be arched back as much as physically possible, and that routine had to be ingrained in your mind. It was important because you had to flex your back, extending it to the max, and hold it for the ten-second, free-fall count. It looked like an exaggerated swan dive. This was the one aspect that had to be practiced repeatedly. They gave us an exercise to practice several times throughout the day, not only at the school setting but also anywhere else we could, as well as at home in the evening.

Position yourself on your stomach on the floor or on a bench. Spread your arms out from your sides until they are near 90 degrees from your body, and then raise your chest and shoulders upward by pulling your head up and back as hard as you can. At the same time, raise your feet, knees, and legs off the floor. You end up almost in a U shape with just the front of your hips touching the floor or bench. That position flexes the paraspinal muscles, those muscles that extend up each side of your spine. As you hold that position as long as you can, those muscles are actually lifting the weight of your chest and legs off the floor.

If you perform that exercise every day, those muscles will strengthen, just like you strengthen your biceps by flexing them as you bend your elbow while lifting the weights in your hand. You will be glad you prepared your back muscles if you ever do a first jump and your parachute doesn't open. You will need to hold, locked into that position, while you find your emergency pull cord and pull with all your might. That is why I know this exercise works on your back. My chute didn't open on my first jump. I have often wondered who the "trusted expert" was who packed my chute that day.

This back exercise is an excellent one to begin practicing. The result will be that you will find yourself walking more upright, back arched properly, better balanced with your shoulders pulled back, and a new gait in your step.

21

Exercising to Prevent Disease

Now let's look at how exercise affects your risk of stroke, dementia, and cancer—as well as how you feel.

Exercise and Stroke

Stroke is the third leading cause of death in the elderly. Such statements relate to death rate, but I remind you again, forget death rate—think about the quality of your life if you survive such a stroke. You can have a light heart attack yet survive to be active again. However, you can have a light stroke and survive yet be impaired the rest of your life. So in addition to the fact that stroke is a leading cause of death, it is also a major cause of mental as well as physical disability as people get older. Don't just think about whether you are going to die earlier or later. Think more of the physical results following a stroke—limping around, being in a wheelchair, having slurred speech, or not being able to use one arm. Stroke may be the third leading cause of death of older adults in the United States, but possibly even worse, stroke is the number one leading cause of adult disability.

A stroke is nothing more than a heart attack in the brain. Eighty percent of arterial blockage results in a heart attack, while 20 percent ends up as a stroke. The same process is going on in the arteries to your brain as in the arteries to your heart. Not only is the same process going on to cause the blockage, but the same prevention is also applicable to both sets of arteries.

The medical journal *Stroke* reports an interesting study of over forty-five thousand men who had no history of disease in the arteries of their hearts or in their brains. Numerous studies had already proven the protective effect of exercise on the arteries of the heart, but this study was set up to evaluate whether exercise had similar protection on the arteries of the brain. These men were examined to see if exercise had anything to do with preventing a stroke. There was a mean follow-up of over nineteen years. What is interesting is that researchers measured the degree of exercise and correlated that with the risk of having a stroke. They wanted to know not only if exercise played a preventive role on having a stroke but also if different amounts of exercise had different effects on preventing a stroke.

The study sought to answer this question: if exercise helps prevent strokes, will more exercise give more protection? Researchers divided the groups into whether they did low amounts of exercise, moderate exercise, or high vigorous exercise. (Your personal exercise program on the Prescription for Life plan will be more aggressive than this study group's, so your numbers should be even better than these reported.)

Their *low* exercise group did essentially no exercise at all, as we refer to it. They described their low exercise group as individuals who were mostly inactive, including reading, watching television, and such. In other words, their low groups were basically sedentary.

Their *moderate* exercise group consisted of individuals who did some type of physical activity for at least four hours a week. This included activity like walking and cycling.

Then those in their *high* exercise group did more than three hours per week of exercise such as running, jogging, or swimming. So theirs is less intense than ours, but you will be able to see the comparison.

Here's what the study found. The high physical activity group had a 31 percent decreased risk of stroke. And the ones in the second group, who did less active exercise, had a 21 percent decreased risk of stroke.

That's a good life insurance policy. Buy it—it's free.

Just to be fair with women, since this study was on men, there are several good review articles showing the importance of exercise in preventing strokes in women. Actually, men should pay attention too, because those studies emphasize the significance of exercise on the arteries of your brain, whether you are a man or a woman.

Here are the results of a ten-year follow-up study presented in the journal *Stroke*. They divided women into groups labeled "no activity," "moderately active," and "most active."

The bottom-line result of the study was that *the risk of dying prematurely decreased as physical activity increased*. Their recommendation was that exercise should be part of a lifestyle for women to prevent strokes.

Here are a few interesting facets of their study. The women who had the highest amount of exercise were leaner and had lower blood pressure. And guess what! The ones in the "most active" group had a slower resting heart rate. (Remember, the slower the resting heart rate, the stronger the heart.) This group had less heart disease and less diabetes.

What can I say? Exercise is an important part of your lifestyle change. What brings this home is the conclusion about the significance of exercise on stroke prevention. When comparing women who did not exercise with those who exercised the most, researches found that the most active women had approximately a 50 percent lower risk of premature death from stroke.

The question coming from these articles is this: how does exercise lower the risk of having a stroke? Another article in the journal *Stroke* probably answers that question as well as any. Researchers pointed out that exercise decreases the process of damage to the arterial walls of the arteries feeding the brain, and they listed two problems that are combated by exercise. One, exercise raises HDL Cholesterol, which carries away excess lethal LDL Cholesterol; and two, exercise helps to lower weight, which in turn also raises the good HDL while lowering the bad LDL. Again, you see the Prescription for Life plan working hand in hand with one strategy aiding another. You get double protection of your arteries, not only from the exercise portion of the plan but also from the associated weight-loss portion. Exercise—lose more weight.

Many studies in the medical literature show that exercise can reduce the risk of stroke by 25 to 30 percent. One such study in the United States showed a 25 percent risk reduction of strokes in general, including both fatal and nonfatal strokes. Another study in Finland showed a 34 percent risk reduction. Plus, researchers in Norway studied *fatal* strokes only, and they found a 53 percent reduced risk of death from a stroke in women who exercised the most.

I will mention one other article, and then we will move on. The article was published in the *Journal of the American*

Medical Association on the risk of stroke in women, as related to the protective effect of physical activity. It stated that physical activity was associated with a substantial reduction of strokes in women. It further pointed out that there was a linear relationship between exercise and fewer strokes, meaning that the greater the activity, the less risk of developing a stroke. The group that exercised the most gained a 29 percent overall reduction in risk for having a stroke, whether or not the strokes that did occur were fatal.

Exercise and Dementia

I personally think this may be the most important section of the whole book. So get focused and let your heart absorb what you are about to read. We have seen how exercise increases the efficiency of your pump, your heart, and how exercise helps prevent strokes. Now we add one more benefit: exercise affects the quality of your thinking and cognitive functions as you add years to your life.

Exercise aids in preventing dementia. Having a stroke is not the only problem arising from blocked arteries in the brain. The same process also results in dementia.

There are two basic types of dementia: vascular and Alzheimer's. The vascular type is caused by the arterial wall problems we have been going over, the LDL Cholesterol splinters getting into the wall of your arteries leading to or inside your brain.

The other type of dementia is called Alzheimer's disease. Some studies show that Alzheimer's is related, in part, to the vascular problems we have been discussing. The basis of the diagnosis of Alzheimer's is in the finding of certain fibers within the brain. That will be covered in more detail later, but right now, know there are things you can do to help prevent both types of dementia.

Here is the important point to remember: clinically, it is difficult to differentiate between vascular dementia and Alzheimer's dementia. You want to do everything possible to prevent either or both from ever developing in your brain. One of those preventive factors is exercise.

Let's see what effect exercise can play on preventing you from developing what many call the "drool factor," where someone sits around in a chair, staring straight ahead, just drooling.

Numerous articles concern exercise and dementia, but one of the most in-depth is an article published in a recent *Journal of the American Medical Association*. It speaks directly to the relationship between exercise and Alzheimer's disease. The study looked at exercise as well as the positive significance of the type of diet we have been discussing.

We will look quickly at the role diet played and then the effects of exercise.

This study followed over eighteen hundred adults for over fourteen years. First, researchers reviewed other studies that showed that a diet high in fruits, vegetables, cereals, and fish resulted in a decreased incidence of Alzheimer's. They gave higher diet scores to the people who ate the most fruits, vegetables, cereals, and fish and lower scores to those eating dairy products and meat. They gave lower scores for eating saturated fat and higher scores for eating monounsaturated fat. By breaking it down so specifically, it is interesting to see exactly what foods affected the development of Alzheimer's. *The Prescription for Life plan eating strategy is substantiated by this study.*

Here are their findings according to the seven food categories. The individuals who did the worst in their Alzheimer's study were the ones who ate the most meat and dairy products, two of the seven categories they tested. The remaining five categories were, as in the Prescription for Life plan, fruits, vegetables, beans, cereals, and fish. The individuals who adhered to the fruit, vegetable, cereal, and fish diet—as compared to the ones who ate the meat and dairy products—had a 40 percent less chance of developing Alzheimer's. That American Medical Association report alone should be a "moment" changer in your life that convinces you never to put into your mouth the foods listed above in the "bad" group—the "picture in your mind" group you learned about earlier. That report is a good summary of what the Prescription for Life plan can do for you.

That initial part of the report, which revealed that what you eat plays a role in developing dementia, is significant on its own. But now let's look at what the study found about the role of exercise. You are going to see a huge impact, which will appreciably encourage you to exercise.

Researchers went into great detail concerning the effect of exercise on dementia. They wanted to see if it was better to do more vigorous exercise and for a longer period of time or if less difficult exercise and for a shorter period of time was equally as good. So many times, you hear that you need to be moving thirty minutes a day, five or six days a week. Others will say that a stroll is all you have to do, or to take the stairs rather than the elevator, or to get out of your chair hourly and take a walk around the office. Researchers set the boundaries for each category for an individual to choose the amount of exercise they performed. This report will help you make an informed decision about the intensity of the exercise you need to be doing to protect you against developing the most dreadful disorder I can think of—dementia.

For vigorous aerobic exercise, they included jogging, playing handball, and similar activities in which you are moving constantly with sustained heart rate elevation. For moderate exercise, they included swimming, bicycling, hiking, and tennis. All these are excellent exercises, but they don't sustain your heart rate elevation as much as vigorous exercise. And for light exercise, they included walking, dancing, bowling, gardening, horseback riding, and golfing. (If they are counting golfing as exercise, I assume the participants were walking and pulling their clubs.)

The bottom line of the study showed that the more physically active the participants were, the lower the risk for developing Alzheimer's. Even for those who were in the light exercise group, it was helpful because the study found a gradual decrease in Alzheimer's as the exercise increased in intensity and length of time. So even if you are just starting out on your exercise lifestyle, you are actually working on improving your chances of not developing dementia.

Here are their results on exercising when they compared the participants who did the most vigorous exercise to those who didn't exercise at all. Listen up to this one.

Those who exercised the most had a 48 percent lower risk for Alzheimer's disease.

There was a gradual decrease of the risk of developing Alzheimer's with a gradual increase of exercise. The more exercise, the more protection.

This next statement is even more exciting. If you include both exercise and eating fruits, vegetables, whole grains, and beans with no meat or dairy, you will be even more protected against Alzheimer's. *The report shows that you can expect around a 60 percent risk reduction with exercise plus diet.* I would vote for that any day, wouldn't you? (Tell all your friends about this report the next time they can't remember someone's name.)

Just take a moment to memorize these numbers from this report: 40, 48, and 60. You get a 40 percent decrease in risk of Alzheimer's with your diet (which matches what the Prescription for Life plan recommends), a 48 percent less risk with exercise, and a 60 percent less risk if you eat right plus exercise. And you know what? If you are doing both of those, I almost guarantee you will automatically get to your ideal weight. Remember the women in the Brown University study? The ones who exercised and dieted lost almost twice the amount of weight as those who only dieted.

Here is one additional point made in this study. Researchers examined a subgroup of older individuals who averaged seventy-seven years of age. They found that, on average, that group didn't exercise as much, but the exercise they did made a significant difference in their health. Some in this group engaged in approximately 1.3 hours a week of vigorous exercise, others 2.4 hours of moderate physical exercise a week, and others 4 hours of light exercise per week—or a combination of the three types. In other words, some may have run some of the time, played tennis some of the time, and even played a round of golf. But the point made is that even relatively small amounts of exercise are associated with a reduction in the risk for developing Alzheimer's. As you age, stick to your strategy of exercise to the fullest physical ability you have.

Even if you are elderly and exercise only once a week, that exercise is beneficial in warding off Alzheimer's. In the early stages of Alzheimer's, an individual's thinking begins to become a little obscure. Their reasoning, their thought process, their rational thinking all begin to change and then just get worse. That is called their cognitive function. In the journal *Neurology*, a study was published that shows older people who exercise at least once a week are 30 percent more likely to maintain their cognitive function than those who don't exercise at all. Defeating dementia is a great bonus most do not even consider when they think about exercising.

Don't forget—exercising is one of the most important things you can do to prevent dementia.

Exercise and Colon Cancer

The benefits of exercise go beyond strengthening the heart and helping to prevent strokes and dementia. The American Institute for Cancer Research reviewed twenty studies concerning the relationship of colon cancer to exercise. Seventeen of those studies found that exercise protects against colon cancer. Their conclusion was stated as follows: "The evidence that physical activity protects against colon cancer is convincing."

Colon cancer is the third leading cancer in both men and women. Let that sink in a minute, because you can do something to prevent being one of those statistics. I had always thought of exercise as improving my heart. But even though I had operated on colon cancer numerous times before, I had never thought much about the effect exercise has on colon cancer. Then I started reading articles like the one just mentioned and realized the positive effect exercise has in protecting against colon cancer.

Exercise and How You Feel

We go from talking about preventing colon cancer to the effect exercise has on how you feel. You don't have to exercise much to realize that you feel better mentally after exercising. That is due to the release of the "feel good" chemical endorphin. Endorphin is released into your body when you exercise. The next time you are feeling low and know you should exercise but are contemplating just sitting down and staring at something, go ahead and exercise and see how you will be lifted up psychologically.

There is an entire section on erectile dysfunction later, but I want to mention here some of the effects exercise has on the problem. A recent study of men forty to seventy-five years old showed that physical activity and physical fitness played a significant role in preventing the dysfunction. The study concluded that the men who exercised regularly were less likely to suffer from erectile dysfunction.

Another article from the *Archives of Internal Medicine* was more specific with the numbers. It stressed two factors related to erectile dysfunction: obesity and exercise. Researchers reported evidence that obesity resulted in a 30 percent higher rate of erectile dysfunction, while exercise was associated with a 30 percent lower risk of the problem.

There is yet another related article in the journal *Urology* concerning men who are in midlife. The study showed that men who initiated physical activity in midlife had a 70 percent reduced risk for developing erectile dysfunction versus the couch potato men—those who were sedentary.

Whenever you exercise, remind yourself of all these beneficial effects your workout has on your body. It not only has a powerful effect on your longevity but also

- enhances your thinking, helping you believe you will succeed on the Prescription for Life plan
- strengthens your heart muscle with an increase in efficiency
- improves your HDL/Total Cholesterol ratio

- helps you lose weight
- decreases your chance of having a stroke
- helps prevent colon cancer
- improves your chances of never having Alzheimer's
- decreases the risk of erectile dysfunction

So are you ready to get started? I'll see you at the gym.

Part 5

Preventing Dementia

The most feared way to spend the final years of life is to have dementia. It can be worse than cancer, worse than a heart attack or stroke. If you are honest with yourself, you are asking if there is anything you can be doing to ward off this dreaded entity.

Most people don't realize steps can be taken to significantly reduce the odds that they will end up sitting in a chair, just staring. There are things you can do to help prevent dementia from ever happening. You are about to learn some numbers from the medical literature that will make you change your lifestyle to give you vibrant, vivacious years as you travel all the way down the road of life. You are about to gain knowledge that will change your thinking—about dementia.

22

What Is Good for the Heart Is Good for the Brain

She always has a smile whenever anyone comes into the room. She sits in her recliner most of the day, and she likes to read, looking at a book at least 80 percent of the time. The problem is that it's the same book and the same page most of the day. She doesn't seem to realize that she is reading the same words over and over. If you give her a magazine, she will turn the pages from front to back. And then repeat the process again and again—until you replace the magazine with the book. She recognizes her caretakers, and her daughter, and me.

But she recognizes very few other visitors.

Her husband, Ervin, has been dead for over eight years now. She will talk to her daughter as if everything is normal, asking her how she is doing and even discussing things that happened years ago. She can remember them vividly. She knows when I was in her home twenty years ago. Even forty years ago. But then she will look toward the door and say that Ervin will be coming home soon. And when it is bedtime, she will say that it is time for her to leave and go home. I explain to her that she is in her home. That this is her living room—and her bedroom is just down the hall. She will look at me with a surprised look and say nothing. Yet five minutes later she repeats that it is getting late and she needs to leave and go home. But now when she says something like that, I simply change the subject and talk to her about the older days, ones she can remember.

Dementia is what her doctor calls it. It is a progressive process. The symptoms started out with her just like the medical books say they do. She began to forget little things. Names . . . where she left her car keys. Then one day she was going to drive to the grocery store but came back home because she couldn't remember why she left the house. They finally had to tell her she couldn't drive anymore. She was infuriated because she knew she could still drive safely. The only way to protect her was to hide her keys. That infuriated her even more.

Then she got better. At least she didn't ask to drive anymore. I would occasionally visit her, pulling up my chair right beside her recliner. We talked; she laughed. I wanted to remember her that way, because I knew she was a part of me and when she was gone, a part of me would be gone also.

Dementia is a terrible way to spend the last five to ten years of your life. It's difficult to live in an everyday world without any idea of what today really is.

Is there anything you can do to prevent dementia? Or is it just something that happens as you get older? Are there some things you can be doing to put off getting it—to prevent it completely? Let's look at what the medical literature has to say.

First of all, a significant percent of dementia is related to the health of your arteries. The health of the arteries of your heart is directly linked to the cognitive health of your brain. You have been learning what is good for the heart. Now learn what is good for your brain.

The two most common forms of dementia are Alzheimer's disease and vascular dementia, with Alzheimer's disease being the most common. Alzheimer's is known to be a degenerative problem within the brain, whereas vascular dementia is a direct result of diseased arteries in the brain. However, more and more studies are showing an association between arterial disease and Alzheimer's.

We have already discussed Alzheimer's disease in relation to being overweight and to exercise, but now we will focus on Alzheimer's disease as a separate entity. One thing you need to realize about the diagnosis of Alzheimer's is that most doctors will tell you it is very difficult to clinically differentiate between vascular dementia and Alzheimer's dementia. Much of what is today termed Alzheimer's is actually secondary to vascular problems of vascular dementia. Many times, the problem is not one or the other but a combination of both.

If you look at Alzheimer's dementia as an individual diagnosis, it accounts for around 65 percent of cases of mental impairment in elderly people. They get to a point where they can't remember things, have difficulty reasoning, may have trouble getting around, and may even end up bedridden, staring at the ceiling. The prevalence of this dementia doubles every five years after the age of sixty, and here is the scary number: it is found in up to 40 percent of those eighty-five years and older. We are discussing serious terms about everybody's future here.

True Alzheimer's is associated with having an unusual type of protein found within the tissues of the brain. You remember our earlier discussion of the importance of eating foods high in omega-3 fat (such as fish, nuts, and olive oil) as a protection against Alzheimer's. Beta-amyloid protein plays a significant role in the findings of changes in the brains of people who are developing Alzheimer's. If the brain tissue is studied, fibers are found made up of what is called amyloid protein. Little nerve fiber tangles are also found in the brain tissue. Studies have shown that people who have higher levels of beta-amyloid in their blood develop Alzheimer's more frequently than those who don't have beta-amyloid floating around in their blood.

So if you took someone who had dementia and found deposits of beta-amyloid protein in their brain, you would diagnosis their dementia as Alzheimer's. But other studies point out that it is not all that simple to differentiate between Alzheimer's dementia and vascular dementia.

How can dementia be prevented?

There is a correlation between dementia and being overweight or obese. In an eighteen-year follow-up study of overweight patients, the women in the study who developed dementia had a higher BMI than the women who did not develop dementia. Other studies found that the risk of developing dementia is greatly increased in individuals who are overweight or obese.

Dementia is not the result of just one factor. The same lifestyles that lead to disease of your heart also lead to dementia. The same precautions to protect your heart help in the prevention of dementia. It is all woven together.

Let me go over a significant study called the Rotterdam Study, which helps tie it all together. This is a study with almost nine thousand participants in which researchers evaluated the dietary fat intake of each group and the relationship of dietary fat intake to dementia. The study's basis was related to the known fact that a diet high in saturated fat and cholesterol elevates LDL and has been consistently associated with an increased risk of cardiovascular disease. The question was, If dietary fat intake increases risk to your heart, does it also increase the risk of developing dementia?

Their conclusion was that cardiovascular disease *is* related to dementia.

This study suggested that a diet high in saturated fat and dietary cholesterol raises the risk of dementia, especially vascular dementia. Plus, they concluded that eating fish may reduce the risk of dementia, including Alzheimer's disease.

At one time there was a medical distinction between Alzheimer's dementia and vascular dementia, but that distinction is fading in many circumstances. It is not one or the other as much as there is a big overlap between the two types of dementia. When the brains of patients who died after a diagnosis of dementia are studied, finding pure Alzheimer's dementia or pure vascular dementia is rare. Most people have at least some component of both.

I'll give you a quick rundown on both types of dementia, but remember, they can be difficult to differentiate and the two can be mixed. Learn how to prevent any type of dementia, whether it is isolated or mixed, and develop your lifestyle accordingly to prevent it.

Certain findings under the microscope are used to differentiate between the two types of dementia. Finding amyloid plaques and tangles with connective tissue has been the main factor used to label someone's dementia Alzheimer's. However, some patients with dementia do not have this amyloid substance in their brains but do have signs of small, multiple, silent strokes caused by the artery problems we have been discussing. These patients have been assumed to have Alzheimer's because the symptoms are so similar.

What I want you to understand is the fact that the two types of dementia are not necessarily completely unrelated. For the brain to function properly, it is dependent on one primary factor: an efficient circulatory system. That is why studies are showing that at least some Alzheimer's dementia may actually be the result of chronic low perfusion of the brain. Some who have been diagnosed with Alzheimer's have had "silent strokes" occur without any symptoms.

It is reported that the arterial changes you have been studying is present, to some degree, in 100 percent of the population in America by age eighty-five. Such reports are revealing the possibility that chronic or transient blockage of the blood flow to the brain may well contribute to the accumulation of the amyloid deposits that are commonly seen in pure Alzheimer's disease.

The large Rotterdam Study mentioned previously evaluated the severity of the arterial disease as correlated with the severity of Alzheimer's, and what they found makes a great point in the interrelationship of the damaged arterial walls and Alzheimer's. The finding is one of the most significant warnings you have concerning protecting your arteries with your new lifestyle. They found that the severity of both Alzheimer's dementia and vascular dementia correlated significantly with the severity of the arterial wall involvement. Their conclusion: *the more severe your arterial wall damage, the more severe the dementia.*

The exciting conclusion is that you are able to do something to help prevent the "drool factor" later in life. The Prescription for Life plan is key in learning how to protect against the damage to your arteries that brings on dementia.

Learn the steps you can take to keep your mind alert as the years go ticking by. Never forget those 40, 48, and 60 numbers. (You memorized them already—remember?) Forty percent reduced risk by eating properly. Forty-eight percent reduced risk by exercising. Sixty percent reduced risk by doing both. And you have learned the details of what to do with the Prescription for Life plan.

Remember . . .

You *can* do something to prevent dementia

You *can* prevent damage to the walls of your arteries

For your mind's sake . . .

Change your eating strategy

Change your strategy for exercise

Change your strategy for sustaining your ideal weight for the rest of your life

If you don't, you may be the one who ends up sitting in your recliner most of the day, always smiling whenever anyone comes into the room, and looking at a book at least 80 percent of the time. The problem is it will be the same book and the same page most of the day. For some preventable reason, you won't seem to realize that you are reading the same words over and over. It *was* preventable, but it is too late at that point.

The truth is, it is still preventable now—by doing all you can to protect your arteries.

Part 6

Preventing Cancer

The biggest fear most people have is dying from cancer. I have been asked many times if a cure for cancer is being developed.

Almost everyone knows the majority of lung cancers can be prevented by not smoking. However, very few realize that *up to 38 percent of breast cancers and up to 45 percent of intestinal cancers can be prevented by developing a healthy lifestyle.* And many women with breast cancer in one breast want to know if there is anything they can do to prevent it from happening in the opposite breast.

There are definite steps you can take to help prevent a malignancy, but very few know what they are. Lifestyle changes are significant for prevention, yet they are not recognized as such. You are about to discover specific steps you can take to avoid dying from your biggest fear—cancer.

23

The Prescription for Life Plan and Cancer

When I researched the three strategies that protect us against aging, I discovered a real serendipity jewel. The more I reviewed the medical literature, the more I discovered that these very same three lifestyle changes also protect us against the most lethal cancers we can develop. It has been estimated that about a third of cancer deaths can be prevented by eating properly, losing excess weight, and exercising. The American Cancer Society's Nutrition and Physical Activity Guidelines emphasize the importance of the three focuses of the Prescription for Life plan in reducing your risk of cancer.

I read in the *Journal of the American Medical Association* that women who lost 22 pounds after menopause reduced their risk of developing breast cancer by 45 percent. It also stated that women who gained more than 55 pounds after age eighteen had a 45 percent increased risk of developing breast cancer as compared to women who maintained their weight.

The more I read, the more reason I found to encourage people to develop a proper lifestyle. One example was finding that *exercise is associated with a 20 to 30 percent reduction in the risk of colon cancer.*

Studies also show that exercise reduces the risk of breast cancer. Women who exercise for about thirty minutes three or four times a week *decrease their breast cancer risk by about 25 percent.* It is exciting to find that the proper lifestyle to protect your arteries to stay younger is the same lifestyle that helps in the prevention of some of our most common cancers.

The American Cancer Society says that scientific evidence suggests that one-third of cancer deaths are related to being overweight or obese, physical inactivity, and an improper eating lifestyle. All three factors are the ones covered in the Prescription for Life plan. They go on to say that only approximately 5 percent of cancers are strongly hereditary. So if you want to blame something for cancer, don't blame it on your genes. Blame it on yourself.

Cancer is the second leading cause of death in the United States. One out of two American males and one out of three American females will be diagnosed with cancer sometime in their life. The three most common cancers causing death in men are lung, prostate, and colon. The three most common for women are lung, breast, and colon.

Here is the serendipity finding: the lifestyle that protects you against heart attacks, strokes, dementia, and other problems caused by poor health of your arteries also helps prevent some of the most common cancers men and women get. That is what the Prescription for Life plan includes with absolutely no extra work. It's like a free bonus.

Listen up a minute. Overall, about a third of the cancer cases reported every year in the United States could be prevented through lifestyle changes that include what you eat, what you don't eat, what you don't drink, not smoking, getting to an ideal weight, and exercise.

In the United States, overweight and obesity contribute to 14 to 20 percent of all cancer-related mortality.

Physical activity is associated with a 20 to 30 percent reduction in the risk of colon cancer.

Physical activity, especially vigorous activity, reduces the risk of breast cancer.

Strategies That Protect against Cancer

An interesting study followed cancer survivors for seven years. Looking specifically at later causes of death, the findings answer the question each one of the patients asked themselves after the initial treatments and operations: "Even though I have initially survived, will my cancer cause my death sometime down the road?"

And if you're a cancer survivor, you may be asking yourself, "Will I die from that cancer or will I die from 'something else'? And if I have survived the cancer, can that 'something else' be prevented?"

There would be nothing worse than to beat cancer and then get defeated by something other than the cancer—especially if that something other was preventable. The cancer survivors in this particular study had the most prevalent cancers men and women get: lung, breast, prostate, and colon. The question the study raised was, Did they die from their cancer or something else? Here are their numbers: 51 percent died from their cancer, but 49 percent died from something else.

Now listen to this next statistic: two-thirds of those who didn't die from their cancer died from heart disease.

The sad part of this story is that the damage to the arteries in their heart was *preventable*! If you have gone through the furnace of being treated for cancer and come out of it, begin thinking of the benefits a proper lifestyle can offer you for the extra days you have been given. Follow the steps of the Prescription for Life plan—getting regular exercise, eating the right foods, avoiding the wrong foods, and sustaining an ideal weight, as well as not smoking.

The big question in everyone's mind pertains to what can be done to prevent cancer from ever developing. The American Cancer Society has some recommendations about what can be done to do this. Here are their current recommendations concerning nutrition and physical activity as preventive measures.

1. Maintain a Healthy Body Weight

It would be nice to be able to turn the clock back ten years and get to your ideal weight, but you can't. What you can do, though, is control it from now on.

The American Cancer Society goes on to suggest that *maintaining a healthy body weight may be the single most important factor you can control to prevent cancer*. That is a huge statement. If you are overweight, you are not doing all you can to prevent cancer. If you narrow the reports down to breast and colon cancer, it gets even more specific. The World Cancer Research Fund and the American Institute for Cancer Research's final report states this: *the evidence for body fatness causing postmenopausal breast cancer is convincing*. It also points out that obesity carries with it an increased risk factor of 25 percent for colon cancer.

2. Engage in Physical Activity

Do you see the similarity in these recommendations and the Prescription for Life plan? Eating properly and being at an ideal weight are important, but exercise is so significant. Exercise is associated with a significant reduction of risk for both colon and breast cancers. To put it in even better perspective, a large study of over four hundred thousand participants found that the risk for colon cancer could be lowered by 20 to 25 percent by vigorous exercise an hour a day.

Add to that the conclusion of the World Cancer Research Fund and the American Institute for Cancer Research: "The evidence that physical activity protects against colon cancer is convincing." If we switch from colon cancer—one of the major cancers in both men and women—to breast cancer, another study on women who had breast cancer shows there was protection against recurrent disease when breast cancer survivors did moderate exercise thirty minutes a day, five days per week.

Another report is from researchers at the University of North Carolina at Chapel Hill who studied over three thousand women, about half of whom had breast cancer. They found that women who exercised had a reduced risk of developing breast cancer. There was a direct correlation between the amount of exercise and the protection against developing breast cancer, but even those who did only daily brisk walking had a reduced risk. Those who exercised more intensely—ten to nineteen hours a week—had the greatest benefit of *almost a 30 percent reduced risk of developing breast cancer*. That doesn't mean you have to exercise ten hours a week to get a protective benefit, but it does say that the more you do, the better, though even light exercise is shown to be beneficial.

What is exciting is that no matter how old or young you are, exercise is important, especially when you focus on breast cancer. Around forty-eight thousand women are diagnosed with breast cancer every year, and 80 percent of those are over fifty. By the time they reach fifty, most women are pretty well set in their lifestyles. So many have not been active, haven't exercised regularly, and don't see any reason to begin now. However, these reports reveal that even if you haven't been active throughout your life, you can still reap the benefit of protection against breast cancer by beginning to exercise at whatever age you are.

Even if you are overweight or obese, exercise plays a role in breast cancer prevention. Medical reports show in studies of overweight females that women who were overweight or obese to begin with and began exercising regularly had a lower risk of breast cancer than those who did not exercise.

3. Eat a Healthy Diet with an Emphasis on Plant Food Sources

Can you imagine a course that teaches you what to eat and not to eat to help prevent cancer? This is it. Do you remember the discussion on red meat and how the saturated fat in red meat elevates your LDL Cholesterol? *There is also a cause-effect relationship between red meat and colon cancer.* Plus, when the American Cancer Society emphasizes plant food sources, that is where fruits and vegetables come into play. That's the Prescription for Life plan. The same plan that helps you stay as young as possible physiologically by protecting your arteries is the lifestyle the American Cancer Society stresses to prevent the most common cancers. You are getting a two-for-one deal with the program.

4. Limit Alcoholic Beverage Consumption

The usual alcohol consumption limit referenced in medical literature is a single glass of wine daily for females and two for males. I remind you, however, that if you look specifically at breast cancer, the recommendation changes somewhat. The World Cancer Research Fund and the American Institute for Cancer Research states that *"the evidence that alcoholic drinks are a cause of breast cancer at all ages is convincing."*

Why This Matters

The first and second ranked enemies you can die from are arterial disease and cancer. Arterial disease causes over 50 percent of deaths, and cancer causes an additional 25 percent. I have stood by the beds of men and women who were dying from each. I'm here to tell you that dying from arterial disease in our hearts and brains is one thing, but dying from cancer is another story. Watching someone go through the valley of death from a cancer can be one of the most horrific events anyone can ever experience.

Being told that you have cancer is one thing. Being told that you have a 50 percent chance of survival means you have a tough road ahead for you, and being told that you have a 20 percent chance of cure makes you pull out all the stops and become willing to put yourself through whatever it takes to give you a chance, even if there is only a slim possibility of cure.

Worst of all is to be told that your cancer is incurable but that the doctors will give you some palliative treatments of radiation and/or chemotherapy, which may slow the rate of growth of your malignancy somewhat. Once you are informed that you have an incurable malignancy, you begin to realize that your time on this earth is more limited than you had thought.

Learn the steps that may prevent you from ever having to go through such a sorrowful time of life.

As a young surgeon, I operated on numerous cancers. I took out lung cancers. I cut out sections of colon for colon cancer. I removed breasts for breast cancer. I thought about preventing lung cancer by not smoking, but I didn't really think much about what to tell patients to do to prevent breast cancer or colon cancer. They just came to me and I operated on them. I knew that in men, lung cancer was number one, with prostate being second and colon cancer third. With women, I realized again that lung cancer was number one, with breast two, and as with men, colon was the third most common.

A few interesting facts are seen in medical literature concerning these cancers. The National Cancer Institute reviewed over three hundred studies that all showed similar statistics—fruits and vegetables are two of the best protectors against cancers, including two of the most common: colon and breast. In addition, there is almost no breast cancer in populations where they consume less than 10 percent of their calories from fat. In these same areas, you don't find obesity. A study from Norway showed a 72 percent lower risk of breast cancer in women who exercised more than four hours a week and who were lean compared to those who didn't fit these criteria.

Now, as an older surgeon, I realize the importance of emphasizing to patients how to prevent lung, breast, or colon cancer. Women need to know that they can help prevent breast cancer by exercising and losing weight. Men and women both should understand that an ideal weight and exercising, as well as eating fiber, will help them prevent colon cancer. That is what I have learned between being a younger doctor and an older doctor. Now you have learned the same.

You can do something to help prevent the most common cancers. You are holding the solution in your hands as you read. I encourage you to do all you can to win the battle against the most common cancers that kill.

24

The Prescription for Life Plan and Breast Cancer

The American Institute for Cancer Research is an international group that reviewed numerous articles on cancer and made a report of their overall observations and recommendations. They are one of the most authoritative reporting councils in the field of cancer.

They made the following pointed observation about breast cancer and alcoholic drinks: alcoholic drinks are a causative factor of breast cancer. This was found to be the case in both pre- and postmenopausal women. The medical literature they studied showed an increased risk with increased intake. That is, the more alcohol intake, the greater the risk of breast cancer. Their conclusion was specific: "The evidence that alcoholic drinks are a cause of premenopausal and postmenopausal breast cancer is convincing."

Many other reports back that up. Recently, an article in the *Journal of the American Medical Association* made a similar observation. This was research done by Brigham and Women's Hospital and Harvard Medical School. It showed that light to moderate alcohol drinkers have an increased risk of breast cancer as compared to women who do not drink beer, wine, or liquor. Even for light drinkers, they found more risk. They pointed out that women who drank only three to six glasses of alcohol per week had a 15 percent higher risk of breast cancer than those who didn't drink at all. And those who drank fourteen glasses a week, or an average of two glasses daily, showed a 51 percent higher risk of breast cancer.

The *Journal of the American Medical Association* did a study of over one hundred thousand women. The study confirmed that women who drink more than nineteen drinks a week have a 51 percent increased risk of developing breast cancer. A single drink was defined as a 4-ounce glass of wine, a 12-ounce can of beer, or 1.5-ounce shot of liquor.

The American Institute for Cancer Research recommends that women not drink alcohol if they want to prevent breast cancer. Another report from the American Cancer Society stresses that, because of the high incidence of breast cancer among American females, risk reduction strategies are essential. They go on stating that "alcohol consumption, even at moderate levels, increases breast cancer risk."

Breast Cancer and Ideal Weight *Plus* Exercise

Being overweight has a direct consequence on increasing your risk of having breast cancer. An American Institute for Cancer Research report found that in postmenopausal women, breast cancer increased with increased body fatness. One interesting observation they made is that if you are overweight throughout your premenopausal years, when you become postmenopausal you are going to have an increased chance of developing breast cancer. They end their discussion by stating, "The evidence that greater body fatness is a cause of postmenopausal breast cancer is convincing."

The reason being overweight has an effect on breast cancer in postmenopausal women is found in research showing that the higher the level of estrogen and some other hormones in a female, the greater the chance of developing breast cancer. Now, this is where the overweight factor fits into the equation—fat tissue boosts the production of estrogen, which in turn fuels many breast cancers. Not only is some estrogen made in fat tissue, but the enzyme that helps in the formation of the estrogen is also stored in the fat cells. So if you have more fat tissue, you are more likely to produce more estrogen, which in turn can lead to a breast tumor. When you lose weight, the level of these enzymes, which assist in forming estrogen, decreases, and you have less of the estrogen to stimulate breast tumors.

The next question that should come to mind is, "If I lose weight, will that in itself cut down on the amount of estrogen, or is there more to it?"

A recent study presented in the *Journal of Clinical Oncology* shows that dropping even a small amount of weight is significant. They found that losing as little as 5 to 10 percent of body weight may reduce a woman's breast cancer risk 25 to 50 percent. The report went on to show that it wasn't just as simple as lowering estrogen alone; inflammation may also play a role in this. They reported that it all goes hand in hand because inflammation is also fueled by fat.

Even more significant was the relationship to exercise. Their study was based on 439 overweight to obese women who did not exercise. Their ages ranged from fifty to seventy-five, and they were randomly placed into one of four groups.

The first group was the "exercise only" group. The study's definition of exercise consisted mainly of brisk walking, along with five forty-five-minute aerobic classes per week.

The second group was the "diet only" group. They reduced intake of fat and calories while increasing their intake of vegetables, fruits, and fiber.

The third group was a combination of the first two and was labeled the "diet plus exercise" group.

The fourth group did "nothing." They stayed sedentary, neither dieting nor exercising.

These four groups of women were studied for a year. They were given a goal of losing 10 percent of their weight. This is where the findings become interesting.

Their blood was measured for levels of estrogen and other hormones. Can you guess who had the greatest drop in weight as well as in estrogen? Can you guess who had the least drop?

Here are the results. By the end of that year of study, the women who were in the diet-only and the diet-plus-exercise groups had met their goal of losing weight. They averaged losing 10 percent of their starting weight. They measured the levels of six hormones related to estrogen. All six are known to have an effect on developing breast cancer. Their findings shine a bright light on the significance of exercising as part of a prevention plan. For each of the hormone levels tested, the women who dieted *plus* exercised decreased their levels significantly more than those in the group who just dieted without the exercise.

Exercise plays a significant role in weight loss as well as in the overall protection against breast cancer. Both groups lost the same amount of weight, but there was a more significant protective factor with the group who exercised in addition to just changing their diet. Exercise was the key. What is most significant in the reviews of the medical literature concerning exercise is that there was a dose-response relationship—the more intense the exercise, the less reported cancer.

A report in the journal *Breast Cancer Research* affirms the importance of exercise. This article found that women who have a family history of breast cancer reduce their risk of breast cancer by a fourth by doing twenty minutes of moderate or vigorous physical activity at least five times a week along with maintaining a healthy lifestyle.

Also, women who have already had breast cancer in one breast were found to have a lower risk of developing a recurrence if they kept at an ideal weight. In essence, getting to an ideal weight represents an additional way to decrease your long-term risk for getting additional breast cancer.

All of these findings simply substantiate the significance of the Prescription for Life plan in protecting your arteries as well as in helping in cancer prevention.

Two things to remember.

First, no matter your age, it's never too early and never too late to make that lifestyle change to reduce your risk for breast cancer. For younger women, it's best to make your decision for the Prescription for Life plan as early as possible so you can avoid the weight gain that creeps up on you as each year goes by. For older women who are postmenopausal and may have gained considerable weight, it's not too late to change your eating lifestyle, to get to your ideal weight, and to begin your exercise program. Bottom line, do whatever it takes to reduce your risk factors for breast cancer.

Second, *nothing good ever comes from being overweight.*

25

The Prescription for Life Plan and Colon Cancer

Do you remember my telling you about those elderly people in Africa and New Guinea who had arteries like a child and had no heart attacks? Cancer of the colon was also unheard-of. That finding is attributable to no red meat intake as well as to their eating a large amount of fiber. I'm not suggesting you move to Africa or buy a gourd to start wearing. Just be aware of what good health is all about.

Colon cancer is the third most common cancer for both men and women. Certain foods play an important role in the prevention of colon cancer, but other foods play an important role in causing colon cancer. Knowing the primary food type that causes colon cancer will most likely cause you to change what you usually eat for dinner. And knowing the food that will give you protection against developing colon cancer will most likely cause you to develop a new eating habit for breakfast.

Contributing Factors

Red Meat

You remember the food picture painted early on in the Prescription for Life plan. (You were supposed to try to forget it. Remember?) That first food on the plate was a steak, representing red meat. Think colon cancer when you envision that picture of a steak on the plate. Many studies show that red meat is a cause of colon cancer.

Alcohol

Alcohol is another causative factor for colon cancer. I take you back to the American Institute for Cancer Research report. They looked at a pooled analysis of more than 475,000 participants who were followed for six to sixteen years and found a 41 percent increased risk for colon cancer in the groups that drank the most alcohol. They found it also to be dose-related, meaning the more alcohol drunk, the greater the risk.

Body Fatness

One more avoidable problem that increases your risk of colon cancer is body fatness. By the way, body fatness reported in medical articles is another term for overweight and obesity. Again, the reports all point out that there *is convincing evidence that being overweight is a cause of colon cancer.* Not only that, but there is what they call "abundant and consistent dose-response relationship" in their findings. What that means is that the heavier the individual, the more the risk of colon cancer.

It should be enlightening to find out that there are things you can do to prevent colon cancer. The good part is that most of what you will be doing to prevent arterial disease also prevents the most common cancers.

You have looked at the negatives that increase the risk for colon cancer. Let's now look at the positives you should be doing to prevent colon cancer. There are two main objectives.

Preventive Actions

Engage in Physical Activity

Most studies conclude that there is a statistically significant decreased risk for colon cancer with exercise. I go back to the American Institute for Cancer Research report because I like the way they word it. They say that there is "abundant evidence" showing a lower risk of colon cancer with higher levels of exercise, as well as with greater frequency and intensity of the exercise. Also, they found evidence of a dose-response effect—the more exercise, the greater the protective effect.

Eat Fiber

Numerous reports show that fiber helps to protect against colon cancer. As a surgeon, I have to tell you that cancer of the colon is one of the worst experiences you could ever go through. So many times, I remember patients coming to me who never had any bowel symptoms at all, and one day they realized there was a bloating sensation in their abdomen. The problem with a cancer in the colon is that it can completely block the intestine to the point where the patient needs an emergency operation. Here is what has to be done so many times in such a situation.

No stool can pass through the blocked area in the colon. The portion of the intestine upstream of the blockage continues attempting to push the intestinal contents through the blocked area. If the blockage is too severe and swollen, many times the only alternative the surgeon has is to resect the part of the colon that contains the cancer causing the blockage and bring out the upstream portion of the colon as a colostomy on the side of the patient's abdomen. Just hearing about this, I would think you would want to do everything possible to prevent colon cancer.

I've made many surgical trips to Africa and New Guinea, where the main diet is fiber. Colon cancer is almost nil around the world wherever fiber is the main source of food. Studies continue to show a decreased risk of colon cancer with an increased intake of fiber. Review in your mind your breakfast menu of high fiber cereal with three of your five fruits for the day, and continue guarding your colon every morning.

26

The Prescription for Life Plan and Lung Cancer

Smoking causes the worst destruction one can do to the human body. Smoking cuts the average life span by about a decade. The *British Medical Journal* sheds light on this statement. It reported a study of seventy thousand Japanese men and women followed for twenty-three years. Men who started smoking at age twenty lived eight fewer years than those who never smoked. Women in the same study structure lived ten fewer years.

Those findings were also reported in a study in *Lancet*, another British medical journal. They concluded, after analyzing the Million Women Study in Britain, *that two-thirds of all female smokers, ages fifty to eighty, die from the effects of their smoking addiction.* Plus, smoking shortened those women's lives by at least ten years.

Time and again, I have had patients who smoked and developed emphysema, lung cancer, or high blood pressure—or had a heart attack—tell me, "If I had only known." If they had only known then how terrible smoking was to their health, they would never have started smoking or would have quit once they realized. But they didn't know. Oh, they had seen reports that it was bad for their health, but they never considered its real consequences for them. They always thought the reports were for someone else who smoked. But now, if you are a smoker, you know.

Here's how bad it can become. I was in surgical training, rotating through the Veteran's Hospital in Lexington, Kentucky. A male veteran in his fifties who had cancer of his larynx, his voice box, was there. He had developed the cancer because he had been a three-pack-a-day smoker most of his life. The picture is still vivid in my mind today. His voice box, his larynx, had been excised, and he was left with a large tracheotomy hole in the front of his neck to breathe through. He could not speak because his vocal cords had been removed with the cancer. His neck hole was as large as if you placed the tip of your index finger on the tip of your thumb. You would end up forming a large zero, the size of his opening.

And that is exactly the way he held his finger and thumb on the front of his neck, over the hole in his trachea. He took the lit cigarette his friend had handed him and held it in the center of the zero—and inhaled. As he exhaled, a steady cloud of smoke came out through the operative site.

Now, that is the most profound picture of addiction you will ever see. If you smoke, acknowledge how bad this is.

Not only does smoking cause 88 percent of lung cancer, but according to an article published in the *Journal of the American Medical Association*, smoking also increases the risk of developing cancer of your colon by 18 percent. If you do get colon cancer, smoking increases your risk of dying from the malignancy by about 25 percent. The colon is a long way from the lungs, but smoking affects your whole body. I made my living operating on patients who smoked. I tried my best to convince people to quit smoking. I spoke at high schools to students to try to persuade them never to start, and if they did smoke, to give it up. I showed students actual blackened, nicotine-stained lungs of patients who had died from smoking. I did everything I could to encourage young people never to take the first puff.

The huge majority of lung cancer is preventable. What about other malignancies? Wouldn't it be a shame to come down with any cancer only to find out later that there were things you could have been doing to help prevent that particular cancer—"If I had only known"? You now know how to cut down tremendously on the development of the most common cancers by altering your lifestyle. The rest is up to you.

With that, we put cancer behind us and move on to a subject most think is for men only. But I want to remind both men and women that there is a hidden lesson waiting. And there is a lot more to it than just erectile dysfunction. It is a warning every wife wants her spouse to know about. So, both men and women, continue reading.

Part 7

Preventing Erectile Dysfunction

There are so many advertisements on television concerning erectile dysfunction you would think 99 percent of males over the age of forty must be affected. Everyone who watches such ads knows the problem, but very few know the actual cause.

If you were to ask the general public what the major cause is, "decreased testosterone" would be the likely answer. But their answer would be completely wrong. If you asked the same crowd if the problem was preventable, most would say no and also be completely wrong. Hardly any of them would know that some dysfunction can even be reversed. But what the general both male and female public does not realize is that there is a hidden danger in a significant percentage of all men who have erectile dysfunction.

This potential wake-up call is essential for every man (and the woman who loves him) to heed. There may be a hidden problem that could be much worse than erectile dysfunction could ever be.

27

The Causes of Erectile Dysfunction

It is important for both men and women to understand the causes of erectile dysfunction. The problem may well be a warning that something much more serious could be going on in a man's body. And wives may be the ones who encourage (okay, nag) their husbands to go to a doctor to get checked concerning something that may be much more serious than a sexual concern.

The most common cause of erectile dysfunction is the partial blockage of the penile artery, with only 20 percent of the problem being caused by low testosterone (which has nothing to do with blockage of the artery).

Erectile dysfunction can be prevented. Sometimes it can be reversed. It is imperative that you understand its cause so today you can begin halting its progress, reversing it, or preventing it.

Erectile dysfunction is much more prevalent than most people think. The Massachusetts Male Aging Study reported that an estimated 52 percent of men, forty to seventy years of age, have erectile dysfunction. They even broke it down to 17 percent being mild, 25 percent moderate, and almost 10 percent severe.

The 52 percent statistic stunned me when I first saw it. I would not have guessed a percentage that high. And then I became more aware of how many television advertisements there are about medications for erectile dysfunction. There are a lot of advertisements, and those ads are directed to only half of the viewing audience.

The same process that causes blockage of the arteries to the heart, which leads to angina, causes erectile dysfunction. The Prescription for Life plan helps in preventing both.

Some recent studies are showing that up to a third of men who have erectile dysfunction already have partial blockage in the arteries in their heart. If you have erectile dysfunction, you—and your wife—should be concerned about the arteries in your heart.

Causes of Erectile Dysfunction

A report in the medical journal *Circulation* titled "Cardiovascular Implications of Erectile Dysfunction" explains the cause well. Blockage of arteries is caused by cholesterol buildup in the blood vessel walls, forming plaques, which make the vessels narrow and slow down blood flow. The article goes on to explain that this blockage process not only affects the arteries of the heart, the brain, and the legs but also has a direct effect on the artery to the penis.

The most important finding they discuss is that this blockage often affects the penile artery first, before it affects the arteries in the heart and the brain. They point out that the penile artery is smaller than the heart arteries or the arteries going to the brain. Basically, what they are saying is that it doesn't take as many LDL Cholesterol splinters to block the small penile artery as it takes to block the larger heart arteries, and you can expect symptoms from penile artery blockage before you would have symptoms from the heart artery.

The medical significance of that last statement is that erectile dysfunction can be a warning sign that there is also blockage building up in the arteries of your heart or brain. Again, they stress the size of arteries. The same process is ongoing in all of the arteries, but these researchers feel that the symptoms show up in the smaller ones first. They are making a point that, because of this progressive order of blockage in the arterial tree, erectile dysfunction may be a warning sign that a heart attack or stroke may be coming unless something is done to stop the development of more blockage.

There may be more than just the size of the artery to this. Perhaps the symptoms of erectile dysfunction do not require as much of a blockage as the symptoms from blockage of the heart arteries. Regardless of the underlying anatomical functioning, symptoms from decreased blood flow in the penile artery many times are a precursor of decreased blood flow to the arteries in the heart.

Think about that just a minute. If you were in charge of setting an alarm somewhere in the body to warn men they may have blockage building up in the arteries of their heart, where would be an ideal place to put that alarm? Placing it somewhere that inhibits sex would get the most significant attention. The message in the medical literature is that there is growing evidence that men with erectile dysfunction should be investigated for disease in the arteries of their heart. Even if you don't have cardiac symptoms, if you have erectile dysfunction, you could still have blockage building up in the arteries of your heart.

To further establish the relationship between the penile artery and the arteries in the heart, the reverse side of the equation is also found to be true. More men with known disease in the arteries of their heart have erectile dysfunction than men who do not have heart disease. One study on two such groups showed that a high percentage of men with disease in their heart arteries also had erectile dysfunction. When this group of men was questioned as to when their erectile dysfunction began, their answers provided astonishing insight. The group of men who had only angina (remember, that is the slight chest pain or discomfort caused from the smaller blockages) said their erectile dysfunction problem began *two to three years* before they had their initial chest pain. When researchers questioned the men who had a full-blown heart attack resulting from a complete blockage of their heart arteries, they said their erectile dysfunction had begun *five years* before their heart attack.

So you can see that the dysfunction can be a warning that you may have angina two years down the road or a full-blown heart attack five years from when your dysfunction began.

Here's the kicker. Protecting your arteries by eliminating the LDL Cholesterol splinters you put into your bloodstream through what you eat, exercising, and getting to an ideal weight all help improve the function of your entire vascular tree. When you protect one part of your arterial tree, you are protecting all of the branches. When you improve blood flow to one area of the tree, you are improving similar flow to the other areas.

The point this article stressed was that if you have erectile dysfunction, *plus* have certain risk factors for developing blockage of the arteries of your heart, you definitely should be checked out for possible disease in your heart arteries, especially if you are under sixty. We will cover those specific risk factors shortly.

Testosterone: Overstated

I mentioned that not all erectile dysfunction is caused by problems with your arteries. Some is caused by a low level of testosterone. You see a lot of advertisements for mail-order testosterone pills as a treatment and cure for erectile dysfunction. If you asked the average man what causes the dysfunction, the overwhelming majority would respond with two words: low testosterone. Just remember that the majority of the time the dysfunction is caused by problems in the artery, while only 20 percent of erectile dysfunction is caused by a low testosterone level.

Let me add one thing here. I had a gentleman patient who had erectile dysfunction as well as two risk factors for heart artery disease—he was overweight and had elevated cholesterol. He had a slightly decreased level of testosterone, and his doctor started him on a testosterone supplement. His erectile dysfunction didn't improve, and the gentleman was at his wit's end about what to do.

If you are like him, just listen up for the next few minutes about things you may want to have checked and do. You want to know your lipid profile, which includes all the cholesterol numbers we've talked about. Your doctor will probably also draw blood for a fasting glucose. An elevation of sugar in your blood can cause damage to the arterial lining, which in turn lets more LDL Cholesterol penetrate into the walls of the arteries. And your doctor will check your blood pressure, because if it is elevated, your heart arteries could be affected down the road as more LDL Cholesterol is pounded into the walls. So, all in all, if you go to your physician and ask to be checked, these are some of the more common tests that will likely be ordered. Any abnormality in these tests may be a heads-up for the possibility of disease of the arteries in your heart, brain, or penis.

Some of the recommendations in medical journals suggest that if you have erectile dysfunction *plus* any risk factors for heart disease, you may need a stress test and other studies to see if you actually have evidence of blockage in your heart arteries. The risk factors include smoking, obesity with a sedentary lifestyle, diabetes, elevated cholesterol numbers, and elevated blood pressure.

28

What Is Good for Your Heart Is Good for Erectile Dysfunction

The same medical literature shows that *weight loss and physical activity improve erectile dysfunction*, that they are key actions you can take to improve your arteries. The Prescription for Life plan not only helps prevent heart disease but also helps prevent erectile dysfunction. And equally important, it can help prevent further worsening of your heart disease as well as further worsening of your erectile dysfunction.

One very interesting study done in England took two groups of men, one from a clinic that was treating men with known disease of their cardiac arteries. They had had heart attacks or chest pain or had to have stents placed in their heart arteries. Everyone in this first group was in a cardiac rehab program, being educated and treated for heart disease. The men in the second group were similar in age to those in the first group, but were being seen for illness other than with their hearts.

So group one had known disease of the arteries in their hearts, and group two did not have any history of heart problems. Both groups were asked if they had erectile dysfunction and, if so, how severe it was.

The finding showed that the group with known heart disease had the most erectile dysfunction. The unique part of this study is that they found out *why* group one had more dysfunction than the men who didn't have heart problems.

Here are the numbers. Sixty-six percent of group one with known blockage of their arteries in their hearts reported that they had erectile dysfunction. In group two, the ones who had no heart problems, only 37 percent had erectile dysfunction. Both groups had erectile dysfunction, but almost twice as many had it in the group with the known bad heart arteries than in the group without heart problems.

The interesting part of the study is that they compared the duration of the erectile dysfunction within the two groups. In the group with known heart problems, the erectile dysfunction had begun five years before they had their heart symptoms. And on top of that, they reported that once they had their heart attack or angina, the erectile dysfunction became significantly worse. The dysfunction went from moderate to severe, as reported in the study.

The conclusion of the study, which was titled "The Temporal Relationship between Erectile Dysfunction and Cardiovascular Disease," showed that *erectile dysfunction may precede a heart event by as much as five years*. That is a great warning statistic to implant in your mind: if you have erectile dysfunction, potentially something could happen to your heart within five years down the road.

Anyone who has erectile dysfunction should begin developing strategies for eating the proper food, getting to an ideal weight, and having a personal exercise program. The reason I say "anyone who has erectile dysfunction" rather than "anyone who has erectile dysfunction plus has any of the risk factors recently mentioned for cardiac disease" is that this study predicts that a significant number of the men in the second group who had the dysfunction but no known cardiac disease will develop cardiac problems within the next five years.

One step further: this study should awaken you to the realization that if you don't have erectile dysfunction or cardiac problems and do not want to have them in the future, you should get started on preventing either from happening.

Erectile Dysfunction and Heart Attacks

Someone with erectile dysfunction is almost twice as likely to die from a heart attack as someone without the problem. I'll give you the actual numbers.

A medical study focused on fifteen hundred men who had no heart problems when the study began. They were divided into two groups, one with men who already had erectile dysfunction when the study began, and one with men who did not. The death rate of the men who had erectile dysfunction was 11.3 percent compared to only 5.6 percent for the men who had only mild or no erectile problems when the study began. This is why you need to realize you are not just talking about a sex problem but are talking about life and death—arterial problems. It's not just about the penile artery not being able to get enough blood flow into tissue to cause an erection; the problem can be a red flag, warning there could be partial blockage in the arteries of your heart.

So often the first symptom of any heart disease is a heart attack, which many times proves fatal. It would be helpful if some alarm could go off to warn of the attack—especially if the person could do something to prevent the heart attack completely. Erectile dysfunction is that alarm in a significant number of men. It is an alarm that informs them they can change their lifestyle to help prevent that initial heart attack from ever taking place.

Many studies show that the more severe the erectile dysfunction, the worse the cardiovascular disease. They show a stepwise increase in risk of heart arterial disease in direct proportion to the severity of the erectile dysfunction. In other words, the worse the erectile dysfunction, the worse the arteries of the heart were.

Erectile dysfunction *plus* known heart risk factors equals an urgency for a lifestyle change to the Prescription for Life plan. Anyone with such a combination should visit a cardiologist for a complete evaluation of your coronary arteries. I say that in all earnestness, because if evidence of arterial blockage is detected early and treated aggressively with lifestyle changes and possibly even medication as an adjunct, many vivacious years can be added to your life. I like to reason that men with erectile dysfunction plus the risk factors of smoking, obesity with a sedentary lifestyle, diabetes, elevated cholesterol numbers, or elevated blood pressure should be considered as having coronary artery problems until proven otherwise.

29

The Prescription for Life Plan and Erectile Dysfunction

I want to challenge you to think about lifestyle changes rather than medication for erectile dysfunction. There are so many advertisements on television for different drugs for treatment of the problem, but three-fourths of the advertising time is spent telling you the dangers and possible harms involved in taking the medication. You need to have an understanding of how the medication works as well as possible side effects of the drugs.

The medication that widens the inside diameter of the penile artery is similar to medicine that dilates the arteries of the heart. To understand how the medicine works, you need to understand what the word *dilate* means in relation to your arteries.

Look at it this way. Let's say that within the wall of an artery there are numerous bands of elastic fibrous tissue similar to multiple rubber bands around the artery. Let's also say that these elastic fibers stay fairly tight and that with each heartbeat they stretch just a little to keep the artery from bulging out too much. As they relax and stretch, the inside diameter of the artery becomes larger and balloons out, like going from a narrow straw to a wider straw. That relaxation allows the artery to open up to let more blood flow through. For an artery to "dilate" is this relaxation of the walls to let it expand in size from a narrow straw to a wider straw. That is what the medications you see advertised on television do; they allow the artery to dilate to let more blood flow through.

If someone feels chest pain—angina—there is medication that can be taken immediately to dilate the arteries in the heart. Once the medication is taken, the arteries expand and go from a narrow straw to a wider one. There is comparable medication that will similarly dilate the penile artery to allow more blood flow needed for an erection. These are the medicines you see advertised on television. There is a direct correlation to the process when talking about angina, heart attacks, strokes—and erectile dysfunction.

I am going to tell you the best story I know to illustrate how medication works on arteries, whether it is a heart artery or a penile artery. There is a pill specifically for the heart arteries, not the penile artery, but both arteries react similarly. The medication is called nitroglycerine. Many people who have known blockage of the arteries in their heart have been prescribed this pill so if they feel a tightness or a pain in their chest, they can place it under their tongue to be quickly absorbed. That pill gives the effect of causing those elastic fibers in the wall of their arteries to relax and allow a greater blood flow, at least for a while longer. I say a while longer because the medication is only temporary and more has to be given, either under the tongue or through a vein if the chest pain symptoms persist.

A few years ago, I was on the initial leg of a six-week trip and traveling from New York to London to Africa on an overnight flight. About three hours into the trip, I was awakened by an announcement overhead, asking if there was a doctor onboard. I went forward and was informed that a gentleman had grabbed his chest and then passed out. He was wearing a suit, and he still had his coat on. His tie and white dress shirt seemed proper for being in first class. And even his handkerchief was still in the top front pocket as I quickly laid him out across the first five middle seats in coach. I immediately asked for oxygen and also if there was any kind of heart monitor, blood pressure cuff, or emergency medication. No was the answer to all my questions, except for the oxygen.

I requested that the crew ask over the speaker system if anyone onboard had any nitroglycerine tablets. Three passengers had some because of problems with occasional chest pain. We had gotten my new patient's coat and tie off, and I had unfastened the top button of his shirt. His pulse was erratic and barely palpable. I kept my fingers on his pulse, kept the oxygen flowing full force, and began placing the nitro tablets beneath his tongue. As soon as one was absorbed, I would place another.

The pilot came back and said, "We are ten minutes from the halfway point of the trip," and asked if it would be better to continue to London or turn the plane around. I said the sooner we got the gentleman on the ground, the greater the chance of saving his life. My reasoning was that if we turned around now, we would get him on the ground twenty minutes sooner because we were still ten minutes before the halfway point, plus getting to the same distance on the other side of the halfway mark would take an additional ten minutes. The pilot didn't say another word but immediately turned and went back to the cockpit.

I will never forget looking out the window and seeing the full moon slowly pass by the window as we were making a 180-degree turn to get our patient back on the ground. In about thirty minutes, although he looked lifeless, he regained consciousness. His pulse became steady and stronger. His suit coat was lying on his chest as we rolled him on a stretcher toward the ambulance. He had not said one word, but his eyes were searching, trying to comprehend all that was going on. He kept looking up at me, and just before we reached the back of the ambulance, he said, "Reach in my inside coat pocket and get my business card. I want you to have it." He was the CEO of one of the largest hotels in Las Vegas. He was also a lawyer for a very well-known individual.

It was only after I returned home six weeks later that I received a call from his son, who had learned who I was through the airline. He informed me that my patient survived his heart attack. Even though he had to be operated on, the outcome was successful.

What did the medication do to his heart arteries, and how does that relate to erectile dysfunction? The pills I placed under his tongue allowed the artery that was partially blocked in his heart to dilate and to allow more blood flow for a short period of time. And as long as I kept placing those pills, the artery remained dilated and allowed more blood flow into the heart muscles downstream of the partial blockage.

Similarly, when you take pills for erectile dysfunction, the penile artery dilates as though from a narrow straw to a wider one, allowing more blood to flow into the penile tissue and making an erection happen.

The basic medicines used to treat erectile dysfunction—Viagra, Cialis, Levitra, or similar type drugs—work by letting the artery dilate to allow more blood flow, similar to what happened to the arteries in the heart of the man on the plane.

The real question you should be asking yourself is this: are there lifestyle changes that will do the same thing?

How to Prevent or Reverse Erectile Dysfunction

Many reports show that heart disease can be prevented by changing your lifestyle to protect your arteries. Can changing your lifestyle also help prevent erectile dysfunction? Will alleviating those same risk factors to the arteries of your heart also improve or reverse erectile dysfunction? Let's see what the medical literature says.

Being overweight or obese affects erectile dysfunction.

Erectile dysfunction can be improved by getting to your ideal weight.

One study dealt with more than fifteen hundred men who had erectile dysfunction. They were divided into three groups according to their weight. They used BMI (body mass index) to determine in which group each man belonged. In this study, almost 40 percent were considered normal weight according to the BMI range.

The study's findings were twofold. They used a Doppler device and measured blood flow in the penile arteries and found that obese patients had more reduction in their penile blood flow, resulting in more severe erectile dysfunction than those in the normal weight group. In addition, they found that the men of normal weight who also exercised had the least amount of erectile dysfunction. (You may want to read that statement again.)

Another compelling article from the journal *Archives of Internal Medicine* found that *obesity is associated with a 30 percent higher risk of erectile dysfunction.*

Another report from the *Journal of the American Medical Association* found that about one-third of obese men with erectile dysfunction *regained* their sexual function after two years of adopting a healthy lifestyle. Their main emphasis was on exercising and losing weight, similar to the Prescription for Life plan.

Not only is exercising and losing weight important to address erectile dysfunction, but the food you eat while losing weight and beyond is important too.

The Effect of Food on Erectile Dysfunction

A change in diet can improve erectile dysfunction. A study was set up to evaluate if eating certain foods resulted in improvement of the problem. They discovered that an eating lifestyle high in fruits, vegetables, nuts, whole grains, and fish but low in red and processed meat was followed more by men who did not have erectile dysfunction.

Then they took it one step further by studying diabetic men. It is known that men with diabetes have more erectile dysfunction than nondiabetics. Yet, even in these diabetic men, those who ate the closest to this basic list of good foods, similar to the Prescription for Life plan eating strategy, had the least occurrence of erectile dysfunction and were more likely to be sexually active. The particular foods you eat do make a difference.

They also evaluated obese men to see if changing their diet had any effect on erectile dysfunction. They found that the obese men who began eating the healthy diet just mentioned had more improvement in restoring function than the obese men who didn't follow the healthy diet. So even for obese men, eating the right foods showed an improvement in the erectile problem.

Because erectile dysfunction is more common in diabetic men, a similar study was done in which diabetic men recorded how much of the healthy diet they ate. The 555 men, who were thirty-five to seventy years of age, had been diagnosed with diabetes at least six months before but less than ten years and were overweight. This is interesting because they broke it down by how well each man adhered to this eating lifestyle. They found that the diabetic men who stuck closest to eating fruits, vegetables, pasta, peas, legumes, beans, nuts, cereal, salads, fibrous whole grains, chicken, and fish were the least likely to have erectile dysfunction, as compared to the men who did not adhere to this eating lifestyle.

Exercise: The Positive Factor

Medical reports show that exercise plays a significant role in the prevention of erectile dysfunction. The *Archives of Internal Medicine* reports that exercise is associated with a 30 percent lower risk of erectile dysfunction. The same report shows that obesity results in a 30 percent higher rate of the dysfunction.

Get lean and active.

And a last reminder for those who are in midlife and adopt the Prescription for Life plan, an article in the *Journal of Urology* points out that men who initiated physical activity in midlife had a 70 percent reduced risk of developing erectile dysfunction than the couch potato men.

Get an exercise program.

Even if you get off the sofa and start walking only one mile per hour, get started and go from there.

The Significance of Lifestyle

A change in your lifestyle offers protection against erectile dysfunction. If you already have the dysfunction, the same changes can improve or even reverse the problem. There are studies that evaluate the effect of combining the three lifestyles you have been learning in *Prescription for Life*. One of the largest studies, and I think the most significant, is from the *International Journal of Clinical Practice*. It is a conclusive summation study of six separate clinical trials from four countries. What I like about this report is that researchers were strict in scoring whether the dysfunction was mild, moderate, or severe. They also were strict in scoring the improvement of the erectile dysfunction by degrees. They targeted diet, exercise, and weight loss as the three significant factors to evaluate how they collectively affected erectile dysfunction.

First, they found improvement in the dysfunction with the men eating similar foods stressed in *Prescription for Life*.

They also found that exercise was significantly important in reducing the dysfunction. To document this point, men who ran for nearly 90 minutes a week or did more vigorous activity for 180 minutes per week had a 30 percent reduced risk of developing erectile dysfunction.

They also included a study of obese men who had the dysfunction. That study showed that within two years of lifestyle change, about one-third of them fully regained their sexual function.

Probably the most significant part of the study was that men already on medication for their erectile dysfunction had better improvement results with lifestyle changes than they had with the medication.

Final Thoughts

Men can prevent or improve erectile dysfunction. The same aging process that may cause erectile dysfunction involves the entire arterial tree throughout your body. Erectile dysfunction can be an alarm and a reminder that your arteries are the cornerstone for the prevention of aging.

Don't ignore the flashing warning signals of your body. (Review this owner's manual frequently.)

Conclusion

As we come to the end of studying how to live younger longer, I encourage you to review what you have learned. Get with a partner or a group that shares your interest in improving the quality of life. Challenge each other. Hold each other account-able with the specific strategies. Find a mentor to help lead you, and become a mentor for someone else. Set partnership goals concerning your weight and your exercise program. Be a reminder to each other concerning what foods you should be avoiding and what foods you should be eating.

Money can get you many things you may want, but whatever you may buy is no comparison to having a healthy, vibrant body. I have shared a review of the medical literature, explaining in lay terms how to live as young as possible. I hope you understand what really ages you. It is my wish that you have a completely different awareness about the working mechanism of your body, the importance of your heart as a pump, as well as the vessels that carry oxygen and nutrients to every single, miniscule particle of your body. I hope you will focus on your physiological age from now on, no matter what your chronological age happens to be. If you have taken this program to heart and already started working it, I know you are physiologically younger today than when you first began, and I want you to be even younger five years down the road. I hope you keep your commitment to eat the right foods and avoid the wrong ones, to get yourself to an ideal weight and keep it there, and to develop a personal exercise program.

I hope this is the beginning of a great journey, living out a vibrant life for many quality years to come. I want for you—*the best*.

Afterword

I have shared with you my many years of medical experience, beginning with that first day in anatomy class in medical school when I actually had the privilege of holding a human heart in my hands. Countless times I've dissected globs of plaque out of carotid arteries that supply the brain with blood. I had my own *moments* of decision that made me commit to a new lifestyle. I hope this book has inspired you to make a decision to live differently from now on.

As I close, however, I want to share one more part of my medical career with you. I became a physician because I wanted to help treat individuals who had medical problems. I look back and remember all the individuals whose lives I had the privilege to improve or even save. That is the greatest reward a doctor can ever hope to receive.

But in reality, we all know that no matter what lifestyle we develop, no matter how healthy we may eat, no matter what ideal weight we chose, and no matter how strict we are with ourselves in exercising, we are all someday going to pass away from this earth. Everybody is dying. From the moment you were born, you have been dying. Everything that has a beginning has an end.

What then? That is the question I made a habit of asking every cancer patient I treated in my surgical practice. What happens after death? Let me close by telling you what I explained to those patients. I invite you to come into the examining room at my office where I have follow-up visits with cancer patients. I have removed many lung cancers. I have removed cancers from the esophagus, the stomach, and the colon. I have had many one-on-one encounters with cancer patients of all ages. I know by their questions what they have been thinking about. I know by a spouse's statement what they discussed the night before.

They all think about death, the dying process, and they all wonder what happens *forever*—after life as they know it.

At the conclusion of their appointment time, I ask if they would like for me to discuss eternity with them. I do not force any discussion on them. I respect our doctor-patient relationship above all else. I would not say one word further if the patients did not ask me to continue. But every single one of the patients I ever asked that question answered in the affirmative. Perhaps for the first time in their life, the question of what happens after they die has come to the forefront in their minds, once told they have cancer.

Pointing to the door of the examining room, I would ask, "If you were to die this moment and that were the door to heaven and you knocked on the door and it was opened, what could you say that would guarantee you admission?"

Most answered something like, "I sure hope I've done more good than bad."

The one answer I will never forget came from a young man in his early thirties. He had an incurable cancer. My job was to keep him alive for as long as possible and to keep him as pain-free as I could. Knowing all the details concerning his future, it was going to be a sorrowful situation. He was sitting on the end of the examining table with his young wife standing off to his left looking at him.

They had an inexpensive car in the parking lot. The clothes they had on let me know their finances were not that great. By his record, I knew he was a laborer, paid by the hour. Here is his answer to the question as to what he would tell the gatekeeper of heaven, what would guarantee his admission. Almost shyly, with his head bent down a little, he moved his eyes directly toward his wife and muttered something so quietly that I couldn't understand what he said. She slowly nodded her head yes. He swallowed and began telling me the most impressive story I have ever heard about getting into heaven—if it could be done by good deeds.

"It was late one night last January." He began his story while continuing to look at his wife. "Temperature was in the twenties, barely snowing. My wife and I were driving down King Street, just before you get into town. There were no other cars on the road and no one was walking. But then we saw this girl, probably in her early twenties, carrying a baby wrapped up in some covers. Walking on the sidewalk. We drove past her but then decided to pull over and back up to see if she needed a ride home. Once inside the car, she said she didn't have a home. That she was just walking, hoping someone would stop—and help her."

He continued looking at his wife the whole time he's telling me this. "We took her to our home and let them spend the night with us. We had an extra bed. She wasn't married. Didn't have anywhere to stay. Her story was sad. The next morning, we decided to go to the bank. We had about sixteen hundred in savings. We took it out and drove her and her baby to an apartment building where I knew the manager. I gave him the money and said to let her stay there for as long as the money lasted."

He quit talking and looked back down toward the floor. My throat was so tight I couldn't respond. Finally, he looked at me and said, "That's what I would tell them." He looked at his wife and then back at me. "That's what I would say and hope they would let me in."

I wasn't sure how to respond at first. I had heard of many people financially giving over and above what they could afford, but I had never met any real Good Samaritans like this young couple who had given their all without expecting anything in return. I knew that if I were the gatekeeper of heaven, I would certainly wish there was some way that deed would get them in.

I told him I had never heard a better example of someone looking out for a fellow human than the story he'd just told. But I also had to explain that even as good as he and his wife had been, that encounter would not get him into heaven.

I pulled out the prescription pad from my coat pocket and wrote "John 14:6." I signed it before tearing the prescription off and handing it to him. As he took it from me and looked at the reference, I paraphrased the verse for him: "Jesus said, I am the way and the truth and the life. No man comes to the Father except by me." I explained that we are all sinners, and though God does not allow any sin in heaven, he sent his Son, Jesus, to die for our sins. He died on the cross, was buried and resurrected, and is now in heaven. If we accept him as our Savior and invite him into our hearts and repent of our sins, we can be saved and admitted into heaven for eternity. I explained that if he did this, that was the answer to heaven. That is what eternity is all about.

I share this part of my medical career with you because I am interested in your health. I want you to have the healthiest life possible. I want you to enjoy life to its fullest. And when the time comes that you finally think about eternity, I want you to know what I told my cancer patients. I want you to realize that your most prized possession is not your health but your soul.

I want you to live younger longer—and even longer throughout eternity.

Prescription for Life 21-Day Plan

Instructions for Use

The *Prescription for Life 21-Day Plan* is designed for individual use, group study, and workplace wellness programs. Groups are encouraged to implement the 21-Day Plan together as a way to support the efforts of individual participants and have more fun making progress collectively.

To use this guide: Start by reading the suggested selection from *Prescription for Life*. Next, read the summary material, answer the **Questions to Consider**, and complete the **Action Step**.

This plan can be read over a three-week period. Alternatively, the plan can be expanded to cover a longer time period, such as 30 days, by reading the material during the weekdays and skipping the weekends.

Once you've completed the *Prescription for Life 21-Day Plan*, we think you'll agree that you will feel better equipped and empowered to live a longer, healthier life!

Prescription for Life
21-Day Plan Outline

Day 1 What Causes Our Bodies to Age? 323

Day 2 Understanding Your Cholesterol Is Critical 325

Day 3 Myths and Misconceptions about Your
Health 327

Day 4 The Three Lifestyles You Can Control 329

Day 5 Foods You Should Never Eat Again 332

Day 6 Satisfy without the Fry 334

Day 7 The Power of the Ten-Second Rule 336

Day 8 How to Determine Your Ideal Weight 338

Day 9 Set Up a Personal Exercise Plan 340

Day 10 How to Achieve Your New Lifestyle Goals 342

Day 11 The Secret to a Healthy Diet 344

Day 12 Eight Easy Steps to Weight Loss   346

Day 13 How to Beat a Food Addiction   348

Day 14 Build Your Breakfast Platform   350

Day 15 Build Your Lunch Platform   352

Day 16 Build Your Dinner Platform   354

Day 17 How Safe Are Supplements?   356

Day 18 Energize Your Exercise   358

Day 19 What's Good for the Heart Is Good for the Brain   360

Day 20 Answers to Prevent Cancer   362

Day 21 A New Beginning   364

Prescription for Life 21-Day Plan—Action Steps Summary   366

A Special Word from Dr. Furman   368

What Causes Our Bodies to Age?

Read pages 39–44, including the sections *How Blockage Begins* and *Don't Let Your First Symptom be Death*. Then, answer the following questions and complete today's action step.

No matter how hard we may try, the aging process is inevitable. Our goal is to live young physiologically—until we die at an old age chronologically. However, did you know that the primary cause of aging can be stopped in its tracks?

Today's reading reveals how our arteries play a monumental role in the physiological aging of our bodies. The flow of blood through our arteries carries nutrients, oxygen, electrolytes, and other essential elements that keep our body running like a new engine. When arteries become damaged by certain types of cholesterol particles, the walls respond by developing a battlefield to fight those foreign bodies. If the situation worsens, this battle can lead to various types of discomfort, blockage, diseases, and even death.

Fortunately, the *Prescription for Life 21-Day Plan* shows how you can avoid damage to your arteries, slow down the aging process, and enjoy better physical and mental performance—for the rest of your life!

Questions to Consider

1. Based on today's reading, what is the single greatest cause of aging?
2. Why are your arteries considered the key to your overall health?
3. Why is it important to turn back the clock on your body's aging process?

Action Step

a. Review the material from today's reading and make a list of the diseases specifically connected to arterial blockage. In addition, list the other organs and parts of the body that rely upon the health of your arteries.
b. Next, make a list of any family members or friends who have struggled with these conditions. It's important to recognize the patterns in other people that could affect you.

Understanding Your Cholesterol Is Critical

Read pages 56–67. Then, answer the following questions and complete today's action step.

Every car has a dashboard with red warning lights to notify you when there is a problem. Likewise, your cholesterol numbers serve as a warning sign when there is a problem with your health. A study was conducted of over 3,000 individuals who died of blockage in the arteries of their hearts. Those with the lowest total cholesterol numbers had an 8-year longer life expectancy than those with the highest total cholesterol numbers.

Cholesterol has two major components. There is the good "hero" cholesterol called HDL, and there is bad "lethal" cholesterol called LDL. Your goal is to keep excess LDL cholesterol out of your bloodstream, while increasing the HDL. When you reduce the LDL cholesterol that causes blockage in your arteries, your organs are able to function at full capacity.

It's crucial to understand how certain foods cause the "lethal" LDL cholesterol to increase and avoid eating them. In addition, your goal is to increase the "hero" HDL cholesterol with proper exercise and by losing any extra pounds you might be carrying.

Questions to Consider

1. Based on today's reading selection, what does "high cholesterol" actually mean?
2. Why is it just as important to increase the HDL cholesterol count in your bloodstream as it is to reduce your LDL cholesterol count?
3. Why is it harmful to wait until symptoms appear regarding blockage in your arteries?

Action Step

Check the health of your arteries by getting your cholesterol numbers tested. This simple and inexpensive step can be performed at your doctor's office, local clinic, or lab. Take time today to schedule this test. It may prove life-saving. If you've had a cholesterol test performed within the past six months, review those numbers. Record your cholesterol test numbers in the four spaces below, and compare them with the "healthy range" levels listed to the right:

_____: Total Cholesterol— *Healthy range below 200*

_____: LDL Cholesterol— *Healthy range below 100*

_____: HDL Cholesterol— Healthy range above 40 if male, above 50 if female

_____: HDL / Total Cholesterol ratio
—Healthy range below 3.5

Circle any number that falls outside of the healthy range. These are your warning signs!

Day 3

Myths and Misconceptions about Your Health

Read pages 82–86 and page 121. Then, answer the following questions and complete today's action step.

Did you know doctors write over 255 million prescriptions for cholesterol-lowering drugs each year? They are written for one purpose—to help lower LDL cholesterol. This group represents the most widely prescribed group of drugs in America. Sadly, many physicians prescribe drugs to treat patients for a problem, but they don't emphasize what the patient can do to fight the cause of the problem. Don't let yourself get fooled into a false sense of security. Even if you are placed on medicine to lower your cholesterol, treat your diabetes, prevent a heart attack, or lower your blood pressure, there is no pill by itself that is the complete answer.

In addition, beware of the misconception about your genetics and family background in regards to your health. Some people tend to rely on their "good" genes and mistakenly think those factors will prevent problems. On the other hand, some people with genetic problems in their family believe that their medical path is doomed. So, they give up on pursing a lifestyle of health. Don't let these misconceptions trap you.

Here's the key: The genes that you inherit are not nearly as significant as the lifestyle that you lead. Lifestyle trumps genetics. The biggest myth is to believe that you can't change from an unhealthy path to a healthy one. You can always change!

Questions to Consider

1. Which, if any, of the myths or misconceptions in today's reading selection have you mistakenly applied to your health?

2. Have you heard someone suggest taking an aspirin a day for your heart? Why does *Prescription for Life* caution against this advice, unless specifically prescribed by your doctor?

3. How does the information you read about genetics change the way you view your health and family history?

Action Step

Write down a medical myth or misconception about cholesterol drugs or genetics that you have believed. Scratch a line through it. Replace it with a statement or statistic that confirms a more accurate reality.

Day 4

The Three Lifestyles
You Can Control

Read pages 26–32, including the sections *Decisive Moments* and *Putting It All Together.* Then, answer the following questions and complete today's action step.

The Prescription for Life plan describes three vital lifestyles that everyone can control. These lifestyle paths determine the destination of our health, play a significant role in our life expectancy, and affect the quality of life that we experience.

Lifestyle 1: Maintaining Your Ideal Weight

Did you know that there is a direct correlation with being overweight and dying from heart disease? In addition, the American Cancer Society suggests that maintaining a healthy body weight may be the single most important factor you can control in the prevention of cancer.

Lifestyle 2: Proper Exercise

Being sedentary can be just as bad as having diabetes, smoking, or suffering from high blood pressure. Yet, over half of Americans are completely sedentary. Performing a brisk walk for just 30 minutes a day, five days a week is beneficial. Consider that if you can't walk a quarter-mile in five minutes, then you are 30 times more likely to die within the next three years than someone who can!

Lifestyle 3: Eating Right

The LDL cholesterol that damages your arteries is based on harmful foods that you eat. We will soon discuss six foods you should never eat again and why. In addition, we will examine the foods that your body needs in order to live the quality of life you desire.

Commitment to the Prescription for Life plan includes all three lifestyles to ensure the youngest physiological age you possibly can have. But remember, the quality of those years is much more important than the number of years!

Questions to Consider

1. Which of the three lifestyles described above do you feel poses the greatest challenge?
2. Do you consider yourself to be active, moderately active, or sedentary?
3. Do you believe that it is possible to give up a certain food forever? Why or why not?

Action Step

Pick one of the three lifestyles (weight, exercise, or eating right) that represents the biggest challenge for you. Use the reading selections listed below in *Prescription for Life* to explore more about improving that area of your life:

- Reaching Your Ideal Weight: Read chapters 13–16
- Eating the Right Foods: Read chapters 7–12
- Getting Proper Exercise: Read chapters 17–21

Day 5

Foods You Should
Never Eat Again

Read pages 131–40. Then, answer the following questions and complete today's action step.

The foods we eat play a major role in our overall health. Because of this importance, there are six types of harmful foods to avoid eating. Let's discuss the first five foods today and cover the sixth type in the next session.

How do you remove the desire to eat harmful foods that seem tasty and fulfilling? Our desires can be changed in three ways. First, educate yourself about the dangers of unhealthy foods. Accurate information can help change our perspective and re-prioritize our long-term well-being over our short-term cravings. Second, replace harmful foods with healthy alternatives that satisfy. Third, employ resolve and willpower to remove harmful foods from your diet.

Prescription for Life has helped numerous people move from "I can't do without this food" to "I don't even miss that food anymore." Sure, you might miss eating a certain food at first, such as donuts or bacon. But, avoiding these unhealthy foods will become easier and easier as you understand the damage that they are doing to your arteries throughout your body. Eating harmful foods can cause you to have a heart attack or a stroke, and even play a significant role in dementia. Improving what you eat will drastically increase the quality of your life—now and in the future!

Questions to Consider

1. According to *Prescription for Life*, what are five of the six foods to avoid eating?
2. Which type of food do you perceive as the most difficult to give up eating?
3. Of all the medical reports discussed in today's reading selection regarding the harmful types of food, which one surprised you the most?

Action Step

Maybe you're thinking, "There's no way that I can give up (insert your favorite) forever." If so, *Prescription for Life* suggests starting with a simple test one day at a time. Pick one of the five harmful foods. Make a commitment to avoid that food for seven days.

Note: If you feel any of the food types discussed represent a food addiction for you, read ahead to Day 13—"How to Beat a Food Addiction."

Satisfy without the Fry

Read pages 141–42. Then, answer the following questions and complete today's action step.

Previously, we discussed five types of food to avoid eating. However, there is one method of food preparation that can turn healthy foods into harmful ones—the process of frying. Fried foods may seem appealing when they're hot, golden brown, and sizzling. But, the picture that *Prescription for Life* paints shows fried food in a different light. There is nothing like a bowl of congealed, dingy-colored grease to remind you that fried foods are damaging to your arteries.

Consider this medical fact when deciding which types of food to eat. One gram of fat contains nine calories, while one gram of sugar or protein contains four calories each. If you eat something fried, you add more calories to your diet. Don't go to the trouble of trying to memorize how many more calories French-fries contain versus a baked potato. Just remember that fries contain a lot more calories than a baked potato. Essentially, the frying process adds about one-third more calories than grilling the same item!

In addition, most fried foods in restaurants are cooked in oil that is high in saturated fat, which elevates your LDL "lethal" cholesterol. In the end, it's easier to learn healthier options and choose to enjoy a variety of meals that "satisfy without the fry."

Questions to Consider

1. What type of fried food do you eat most regularly? Why is it so important to forego this unhealthy option?

2. After completing today's reading selection, what cooking methods does *Prescription for Life* say are healthier than frying?

3. Why are canola oil and olive oil better cooking alternatives than other oils?

Action Step

a. Take a moment to list some of the other ways that restaurants describe fried foods, such as "pan-fried," " battered," etc. Avoid these menu items when ordering out.

b. Prepare some questions that you can ask a waiter, waitress, or cashier when ordering a meal at a restaurant. For example, you can ask, "How is this prepared?" or "Do you have a grilled option?" Practice saying these questions out loud.

The Power of the
Ten-Second Rule

Read pages 124–30. Then, answer the following questions and complete today's action step.

Winning the battle against the aging process begins in the grocery store aisle. You take the first step in defeating your desire to eat unhealthy food when you keep those foods from entering your home. But, how do you pick the right foods at the grocery store? How do you know which food to buy and which food to never place into your cart?

Prescription for Life suggests using the "Ten-Second Rule." It takes only ten seconds to check the Nutrition Facts label that appears on every packaged food in America. You don't need to look at all of the information listed on the label. Just focus on the "bad three" numbers as described in today's reading selection. These three numbers represent the harmful elements in foods that can elevate the LDL "lethal" cholesterol in your blood.

Once you develop the habit of looking at the Nutrition Facts label when shopping at the grocery or convenience store, it will take less than ten seconds to decide whether to put the food in your cart or back on the shelf. Be prepared to see lots of labels with numbers that are completely out of the healthy range. For example, pre-packaged foods, like doughnuts and cakes, are loaded with saturated fat. But, you will also find great food choices that are similar to what you want but have lower saturated fat content. All you need to do is use the "Ten-Second Rule" and look!

Questions to Consider

1. How often do you check Nutrition Facts labels when you shop? Why or why not?

2. Based on *Prescription for Life's* recommendation about examining the Nutrition Facts labels, how do you identify which foods you should never buy?

3. When looking at a Nutrition Facts label while shopping for food, what total amount of saturated fat, trans fat, and dietary cholesterol should be the goal? (For the answer, review pages 129–30 in *Prescription for Life*.)

Action Step

a. Take five minutes today to look at the Nutrition Facts labels on the favorite food items in your pantry and refrigerator. Make note of the items that do not fall into the healthy range recommended in *Prescription for Life*.

b. On your next visit to the grocery store, stop to compare the saturated fat amount listed on a bag of regular potato chips versus the baked chips version. Look for other comparisons of familiar items, such as butter, mayonnaise, salad dressings, etc. Choose items within the *Prescription for Life* recommended range.

Day 8

How to Determine
Your Ideal Weight

Read pages 176–84. Then, answer the following questions and complete today's action step.

In *Prescription for Life*, Dr. Furman cites numerous statistics and medical studies that show nothing good comes from being overweight. In fact, there is a direct correlation between body weight and premature mortality. On the other hand, there are multiple benefits to maintaining an ideal weight, such as the decreased risk of heart disease, cancer, and dementia. Not to mention, you will feel better and more energized at a healthy weight.

Surprisingly, less than 12 percent of Americans are at their ideal weight. Worse, only 2–20 percent of dieters are able to maintain their initial weight loss. Fad diets often contribute to the quick regaining of weight. The Prescription for Life plan focuses on how to sustain your weight loss for the rest of your life. It points out the secret for not regaining weight. This secret is that the eating habits you develop to lose weight are the same habits you use to keep unwanted weight from coming back. Once you reach your ideal weight, you can add snacks and larger portions, but your eating choices will remain the same.

Questions to Consider

1. Using today's reading selection, what is the difference between a "normal" body mass index (BMI) and your ideal weight (see page 176)?
2. What issues do you feel keep you from reaching your ideal weight?
3. How are the penalties of being overweight similar to the dangers of smoking?

Action Step

Besides knowing your cholesterol numbers, determining your ideal weight will give you the truest sense of your overall health. Use the spaces below to begin a record of where you are now and where you want to be regarding your body weight.

a. Current weight: _____
b. Ideal weight: _____

How to Determine Your Ideal Weight

For men, use 105 pounds as a baseline for the first five feet of your height, then add 5 pounds to that baseline for every inch over five feet.

For women, use 95 pounds as a baseline for the first five feet of your height, then add 4 pounds to that baseline for every inch over five feet.

Day 9

Set Up a Personal Exercise Plan

Read pages 228–36, including the sections *Aerobic Exercise* and *Heart Strength Indicator.* Then, answer the following questions and complete today's action step.

Maintaining your ideal weight by diet alone is difficult, which is why exercise is so important. Consider the Brown University study cited in the text, where two groups of overweight women were compared. One group dieted and exercised while the other group only dieted. The women who dieted and exercised lost almost twice the weight as the women who did not exercise.

There are many benefits to exercise beyond just burning calories. Exercise helps lower your blood pressure, strengthens your heart, increases HDL "hero" cholesterol, and reduces the incidence of diabetes, dementia, and even certain cancers!

Dr. Furman recommends that you design your own personal exercise program, because everyone is different physically and different routines may be necessary. However, the main objective is to start exercising today.

Questions to Consider

1. What obstacles prevent you from exercising for 30 minutes a day, 5–6 days a week? Identify the changes you need to make to overcome these obstacles.
2. Why is exercise just as important to raise your HDL "hero" cholesterol as avoiding harmful foods to lower your LDL "lethal" cholesterol?
3. How is having a lower resting heart rate an indicator of your heart's condition?

Action Step

a. Turn to the chart on page 234 and determine your current fitness level.
b. Using the guidelines on page 234, write out a two-week exercise plan What specific activities will you do? What time of day? Begin your plan today.

Day 10

How to Achieve
Your New Lifestyle Goals

Read pages 90–101, including the sections *Case Studies on Commitment* and *How to Get from Here to There*. Then, answer the following questions and complete today's action step.

Today's reading highlights the difference between decision and commitment and explains how taking action is the key to success. Use today as a positive step to reaffirm the commitment you have made to your current and future health. Use these two helpful facts for extra momentum:

- Studies show that people who pre-decide on a goal and write it down are 10–20 times more likely to succeed.
- Accountability and success go hand-in-hand. A recent study showed that people who recruited an accountability partner lost 20 percent more weight than individuals who lost weight without an accountability partner.

Questions to Consider

1. In today's reading, how were you challenged or encouraged by the *Case Studies on Commitment* section that discussed Susie and J.B.?

2. What little things have helped you achieve a goal in the past? In contrast, what little things have sabotaged a goal you pursued in the past?

3. List three ways that having an accountability partner could help you stay on course on the Prescription for Life plan.

Action Step

a. Write down any long-term, intermediate, and short-term action goals for each of the three lifestyle areas: weight, exercise, and eating habits. Use page 98 in *Prescription for Life* as a guide for writing a commitment statement to sign and date.

b. Write your goal weight on a sticky note and place it in a prominent place where you can see it often, such as your wallet, purse, or bathroom mirror.

c. Recruit an accountability partner or support group who will agree to encourage each other to finish the Prescription for Life plan. Write down your goals to show this group. Determine how often you will communicate about your progress. Remember to reinforce the good. But, don't shy away from challenging each other when little things and excuses sabotage your commitment to a longer, healthier life.

Day 11

The Secret to a Healthy Diet

Read pages 146–50, including the sections *Prescription for Life Foods* and *Healthy Choices for Every Meal*. Then, answer the following questions and complete today's action step.

No diet is a success if the weight that was lost soon returns! But, Dr. Furman's secret really helps make a diet successful. He recommends using the same simple eating strategy to lose weight and to keep the weight off. In other words, you make a lifestyle change that you can keep for the rest of your life.

Temporarily going on a diet does not work. Instead, *Prescription for Life* suggests using smaller portions when losing weight and adding between-meal snacks after achieving an ideal weight. Keep the basic rules of what foods to eat and what foods to avoid the same throughout the weight loss process as well as in your weight maintenance plan.

The Prescription for Life plan also recommends focusing on eating healthy foods that you can enjoy. Don't mourn over the foods you give up, especially when those foods contribute to premature deterioration of your arteries and death! Instead, relish in the variety of good food that can be found in a healthy diet consisting of fruits, vegetables, whole grains, peas, legumes,

344

nuts, pasta, and lean proteins, such as fish and chicken. (We will discuss more details about how to structure meals that are enjoyable and satisfying).

Questions to Consider

1. Based on today's reading selection, how many servings of fruits and vegetables are recommended to eat? How many do you currently eat per day?

2. What are four positive changes shared on page 148 in *Prescription for Life* that you can make to your present diet, if necessary?

3. What is the biggest difference in *Prescription for Life's* weight loss plan compared to the quick weight loss plans that you see advertised?

Action Step

a. Review the list below of five healthy food categories that are recommended under the Prescription for Life plan. Write out 2–3 specific kinds of food that you can enjoy eating for each category:
   - Fruits:
   - Vegetables:
   - Whole Grains:
   - Peas, Legumes & Nuts:
   - Lean Meats:

b. Using the five categories above, make a list of healthy foods to purchase on your next trip to the grocery store.

Day 12

Eight Easy Steps to Weight Loss

Read pages 195–204, including the sections *Three Secrets to Losing Weight* and *Eight Easy Steps for Controlling Weight*. Then, answer the following questions and complete today's action step.

Dr. Furman's *Prescription for Life* offers three overarching secrets for losing weight in today's reading selection. Even better, there are eight easy steps that can help you in your weight loss goal, whether you are eating at home or dining out.

Remember this basic principle when choosing what to eat—select the best foods with the fewest calories. The top two options that satisfy hunger with the fewest calories are 1) fruits and 2) vegetables. Choosing these foods may seem easier to some than others. Over time, though, your desire for the foods you think are impossible to do without will decline greatly. Even Dr. Furman remembers days when he didn't think he could give up his favorite food: cheese. But, he made the change and so can you!

In future sessions, the *Prescription for Life 21-Day Plan* will go through a meal-by-meal breakdown. The meal samples, along with the eight easy steps in today's section, will guide you in the decisions you need to make as you work through your diet plan.

Questions to Consider

1. Based on today's reading, which challenge poses the most difficulty to your healthy eating habits?
   - Eating the right foods
   - Avoiding the wrong foods
   - Reducing portion sizes
   - Too much snacking
   - Difficulty ordering healthy food when dining out
2. Why is eating fruits and vegetables the secret to losing weight?
3. How is *Prescription for Life*'s food-focused perspective (see page 199) different than "calorie counting"?

Action Step

a. If you are trying to lose excess weight, unhealthy snacks can sabotage your efforts. Look at the calories listed on the snacks in your home, office, or car. Do any of those snacks need to be thrown out or put away until you reach your weight-loss goal?

b. If you are in weight-loss or weight-maintenance mode, list some strategies for dining out that will help you achieve your goal (for help, see pages 196–204 in *Prescription for Life*).

Day 13

How to Beat a Food Addiction

Read pages 101–7, including the sections *The Ten-Minute Factor* and *A Ten-Minute Success Story.* Then, answer the following questions and complete today's action step.

Beware of diets that say it's okay to eat unhealthy types of food as long as you do so in moderation. The bottom line is that the desire for certain foods is the problem. Moderation won't beat desire. Moderation can get you killed!

If your desire to eat certain foods seems to overpower your self-control, you may have a food addiction. But, you can overcome it if you acknowledge your addiction to harmful foods, such as cookies, ice cream, cheese, red meats, and fried food. Just as with any other type of addiction, you don't taper your consumption—you've got to abstain.

Dr. Furman's experience with patients who are addicted to certain foods has shown that it takes about two months—ten minutes at a time—to substitute a harmful food with a good replacement (see his explanation on pages 101–7 in *Prescription for Life*). He has worked with numerous people who now enjoy new, healthy food in the same way they used to enjoy the old, damaging stuff.

The day can come when you won't care about eating a bite of a harmful food that seems so attractive to you today. Replacing an unhealthy food addiction with good eating habits takes daily sacrifices. But, the results add up to a lifetime of benefits.

Questions to Consider

1. Have you tried to stop eating harmful foods but can't seem to break the habit? Are there any types of unhealthy food that might represent an addiction for you?
2. Based on today's reading, how does a food addiction compare to other types of addiction, such as smoking?
3. If you tried a diet formula that recommended tapering from harmful foods versus abstaining, did you experience long-term success? Why or why not?

Action Step

a. Put the Prescription for Life plan to the test. Write down which foods you are willing to stop eating for two months. Who can you enlist as an accountability partner for support? What will be your reward (not food-related) when you accomplish your goal?
b. As you abstain from unhealthy food, you still need to eat! Based on the information in *Prescription for Life*, make a list of healthy alternatives to replace addictive foods, such as exchanging olive oil for butter, eating fruit instead of a candy bar, etc.
c. Write down three options for activities or distractions that you can do during the ten minutes of self-control time when you forego your addiction.

Day 14

Build Your Breakfast Platform

Read pages 151–54, including the section *Breakfast: The Easiest Platform*. Then, answer the following questions and complete today's action step.

Even if you are in the weight-loss stage, you should eat three meals a day. This is part of a healthy lifestyle. Your day starts with breakfast. Yet, many people choose to skip this meal. However, medical studies show that nearly 80 percent of people who lose weight and keep it off eat breakfast every day. Second, breakfast is the easiest time to get a significant number of the fruits we need daily.

The Prescription for Life plan suggests three basic, platform meals every day for a three-week period. Keep it simple. After the three weeks, you can add a second or third alternate tier to your initial platform. Each breakfast meal should avoid saturated fats, trans fats, and dietary cholesterol.

Your platform diet consists of basic foods that will automatically come to mind when you think of a particular meal. Each platform will consist of a list of foods you will use as a foundation for that particular meal. The rule of thumb in the Prescription for Life plan is to aim for a combination of five fruits and vegetables per day. Breakfast is the easiest meal to set into your new lifestyle because it is so easy to fulfill the necessary servings of fruits.

Breakfast is also the time to put friendly fiber into your day. There are several ways to increase your fiber throughout the day, but breakfast is the simplest and easiest meal in which to get the most total fiber at one time. In the next two sessions, we will discuss the specifics of lunch and dinner platform meals.

Questions to Consider

1. What improvements do you need to make to your typical breakfast meals?
2. What is the most important component when choosing a healthy cereal to eat?
3. Why is fiber so important to good health?

Action Step

Consider the list of breakfast platform meals offered in *Prescription for Life* on pages 151–54. List the options that appeal to you the most and make a breakfast plan for the next seven days.

Day 15

Build Your Lunch Platform

Read pages 155–56, including the section *Lunch: Keep it Simple.* Then, answer the following questions and complete today's action step.

Previously, we discussed how to create a healthy breakfast each day. Let's now look at ways to improve lunch. Remember that the Prescription for Life plan proposes simple meals with no snacks in between if you are trying to lose weight.

As with breakfast, fiber is also your friend at lunch. *Prescription for Life* recommends making vegetables the base of your lunch. For example, salads are an easy way to fit more fruits and vegetables into your diet. They are available everywhere, easy to make at home, and different toppings offer variety enough for every day of the week. Even fast-food restaurants have salads on their menu these days.

Consider other fiber-filled options for lunch, such as a vegetable plate, healthy soups, or a sandwich using grilled chicken or fish. Be sure to check the ingredients and "Nutrition Facts" label of your lunch options to avoid getting sabotaged. Also, choose grilled food instead of fried, and make sure the soup is not cream based. Watch out for fat-laden toppings that make their way onto salad bars and pre-prepared salads. With wise choices, lunch can become one of the most effective meals of your day!

Questions to Consider

1. What are several salad toppings you like that fall within the *Prescription for Life* diet consisting of fruits, vegetables, whole grains, peas, legumes, nuts, fish, or chicken?
2. What two lean protein options does *Prescription for Life* suggest as the best alternatives when you have a desire for meat?
3. What are two items that people usually pour onto a salad can add several hundred calories and lots of saturated fat?

Action Step

Plan seven days of lunches using the guidelines from today's reading in *Prescription for Life*.

Day 16

Build Your Dinner Platform

Read pages 157–58, including the section *Dinner: Developing Variety.* Then, answer the following questions and complete today's action step.

Dinner will depend, to a certain extent, on what you had for lunch. Vegetables are still your primary platform. A vegetable plate is easy to make at home or order in a restaurant. Salad is a good choice for your evening meal as well, especially if you are in the weight-loss part of the plan. A starter salad can also give you extra vegetables while allowing you to eat less of your entrée.

You will develop personal favorites as you develop a basic platform for each meal of the day. But, keep these two things in mind:

(1) Avoid fried foods, red meat, cheese and other dairy products.

These unhealthy foods are listed here again for a reason. Unless you make a decision to avoid such foods, it is easy to let them creep back into your eating lifestyle. They can silently work on your arteries, with you being completely unaware of the damage.

(2) Fruits and vegetables fill you up the most with the fewest calories possible.

This second point is repeated throughout *Prescription for Life* because it is so important. It also flies in the face of the typical American dinner. We are so accustomed to making a large cut of meat the centerpiece of dinner. Instead, try a different tactic. Choose a vegetable or whole grain as the starting point for your meal. Pasta or brown rice bases are good options for your dinner platform. Vegetables and grilled chicken or fish can be added with light sauces if desired.

There is a unique aspect of the *Prescription for Life* strategy for eating. Your platform diet will be the same whether you are losing weight or maintaining your ideal weight. Once you have reached your ideal weight, you can choose foods to add to your basic platforms. The meals we've discussed in the past three days include foods that you might at first have to choose to eat. You will find that you begin wanting to eat them. Eventually, these will become the foods you enjoy!

Questions to Consider

1. What kinds of sauces are approved in the Prescription for Life plan?
2. What is a secondary benefit to eating grilled fish once or twice a week?
3. Based on *Prescription for Life*'s suggestions, how feasible is it to eat well when eating out?

Action Step

Plan seven days of healthy dinners using the guidelines from today's reading in *Prescription for Life*.

Day 17

How Safe Are Supplements?

Read pages 76–81. Then, answer the following questions and complete today's action step.

The Prescription for Life plan is based on the reality that there are no easy alternatives to defeat the aging process. You can't trick your body into becoming healthy. Instead, the proper lifestyle of losing weight, exercising, and eating the right foods is the solution.

Yet, you've probably seen an abundance of well-advertised supplements that promise all kinds of unfounded claims. You may even hear personal testimonies from someone who swears by a particular product. The Prescription for Life plan urges you to beware of supplements. Taking supplements represents one of the greatest senses of false security that Dr. Furman has encountered in his medical career.

Herbal medicines and alternative drugs do not undergo the investigative testing that the national Food and Drug Administration requires. Today's reading shows how important double-blind studies are to protect anyone taking a specific medication. There are many similar situations to the patient's story in *Prescription for Life*, especially related to weight-loss products.

If you are taking any herbal medications, Dr. Furman urges you to consider discontinuing their use. Not just the "medicines" for weight loss, but those that are supposed to make you feel better, increase your energy, improve your overall health, or boost your memory. It may not cause any problem in 99 percent of your friends who are taking it, but you may be the one in a hundred who reacts to the medicine in a permanently damaging way. Beware of the danger of supplements.

Questions to Consider

1. From *Prescription for Life*'s perspective, are there any safe supplements?
2. Are you taking any pill, powder, juice, or substance that is not prescribed by your physician?
3. Before taking any pill not prescribed by your doctor, what questions should you ask about its validity?

Action Step

Remove any medicine, pill, powder, or liquid from your diet that has not been prescribed by your physician.

Day 18

Energize Your Exercise

Read pages 237–42, including the section *Anaerobic Exercise.* Then, answer the following questions and complete today's action step.

Many people view exercise as an activity that burns calories, which results in weight loss. Thus, the focus is on physique or the way our bodies look. While calorie burning is certainly valuable, there are many more benefits from exercise.

However, very few people actually "enjoy" exercise during the moment. It can be difficult to maintain the strain of huffing and puffing for thirty minutes or more. But, there's a hidden benefit to working out. Dedicated exercise helps convince your mind that you're serious about achieving your goals. You intend to stay at an ideal weight. You're going to watch what you eat and don't eat. Consistent exercise helps provide emotional reinforcement.

Additional benefits to exercise include lowering blood pressure, strengthening your heart, and reducing incidence of diabetes, dementia, and certain cancers. Anaerobic exercise is helpful for balance, coordination, agility, and bone density. Keep these long-term benefits in mind to energize your exercise!

Questions to Consider

1. What is the difference between aerobic exercise and anaerobic exercise?
2. Why do people tend to lose strength as they get older?
3. What are some ways you can you perform strength exercises at home, even without special gym equipment?

Action Step:

a. For the next four days, try one of the anaerobic exercises listed for each area of the body: legs, arms, upper body, core, and para-spinal muscles (see pages 238–41 in *Prescription for Life* for details).

b. Using the two-week aerobic exercise plan that you developed on Day 9, what specific anaerobic activities will you add? What time of day is easiest to do these exercises?

Note: For further reading on the different levels of intensity to strive for during exercise, read pages 220–27 in Prescription for Life.

Day 19

What's Good for the Heart Is Good for the Brain

Read pages 257–63. Then, answer the following questions and complete today's action step.

Did you know there are ways to reduce your chance of dementia by up to 60 percent? Suffering a stroke is not the only problem that arises from blocked arteries in the brain. The same problem can also be a significant factor in the cause of dementia. Suffering from dementia is a terrible way to spend the last ten years of your life. This is the average length of time that someone has dementia. But, you can do things that will help prevent it as you get older.

The two most common forms of dementia are Alzheimer's disease and vascular dementia. Your brain needs essential nutrients to function properly. So, your brain tissue will be negatively affected if you block a significant portion of the blood flow to that area. Fortunately, you can prevent this problem through the Prescription for Life plan. What's good for the heart is also good for the brain! Consider the following summary of medical research as reported in *Prescription for Life*. A study

360

of 1,800 adults over fourteen years showed, on the two ends of the spectrum:

- Individuals who did the worst were the ones who ate the most meat and dairy products, while the ones who ate fruits, vegetables, whole grain, nuts and fish, had a 40 percent less chance of developing Alzheimer's.
- The group who exercised the most had a 48 percent lower risk for Alzheimer's disease than the sedentary group.
- The group who exercised the most and ate the proper foods had a 60 percent less change of Alzheimer's than the group who ate the worst and were also sedentary.

Questions to Consider

1. What type of diet raises the risk of dementia? (See page 261.)
2. What is the distinction between vascular dementia and Alzheimer's disease?
3. How important is it to you to stave off the effects of dementia in your old age?

Action Step

Commit the following numbers (40 / 48 / 60) to memory, because they are good for your brain! Memorize them as motivation to pursue a healthier life now and as you age.

- 40 percent reduced risk of dementia by eating properly.
- 48 percent reduced risk of dementia by exercising.
- 60 percent reduced risk of dementia by doing both.

Day 20

Answers to Prevent Cancer

Read pages 267–75, including the sections *Strategies that Protect against Cancer* and *Why This Matters*. Then, answer the following questions and complete today's action step.

The two most common ways that people die are from arterial-related disease and cancer. Arterial disease causes over 50 percent of deaths, and cancer causes an additional 25 percent. Most people know that lung cancers can be prevented by not smoking. However, very few realize that up to 38 percent of breast cancers and up to 45 percent of intestinal cancers can be prevented by developing a healthy lifestyle!

There are definite steps you can take to help prevent a malignancy. These strategies fall right in line with the Prescription for Life plan. For instance, the American Cancer Society states that one-third of cancer cases reported every year in the United States could be prevented through lifestyle changes that include: watching what you eat, what you don't eat, what you don't drink, not smoking, getting to an ideal weight, and exercising.

Sound familiar? These are the same strategies recommended in the Prescription for Life plan. You can dramatically improve the quality of your later years by making wise decisions today.

Consider the following summary of medical reports compiled in *Prescription for Life.*

- The American Institute for Cancer Research showed that red meat is a convincing cause of colon cancer. The same institute found a 41 percent increased risk for colon cancer in the participants who drank the most alcohol.
- Women who exercise around 30 minutes, three or four times a week, can decrease their breast cancer risk by about 25 percent.
- Women who gained 55 pounds after the age of 18 had a 45 percent greater chance of developing breast cancer. Women who lost 5 to 10 percent of their excess weight had a 25 to 50 percent less chance of developing breast cancer.

Questions to Consider

1. How important is it to you to reduce your chances of several types of cancer?
2. Based on today's reading selection, what percent of cancers can be prevented by the lifestyle changes emphasized in *Prescription for Life?*
3. What common beverage mentioned in today's reading selection, contributes to the risk of both breast and colon cancer?

Action Step

Read Dr. Furman's advice on preventing these three cancers in *Prescription for Life:*

Chapter 24: Breast Cancer
Chapter 25: Colon Cancer
Chapter 26: Lung Cancer

A New Beginning

Read pages 108–13, including the sections *Habits: How to Autopilot Life* and *Setting Goals*. Then, answer the following questions and complete today's action step.

The purpose of the Prescription for Life plan is not to give you a list of black-and-white do's and don'ts. It is to inform you so that you can make your own decisions about the direction you are going to take. Remember, your direction determines your destination.

If staying as young as possible comes down to prevention, prevention comes down to one word: commitment. The commitment you have made to educating yourself and taking necessary action steps will build hope and optimism that you are going to be successful in developing your ideal lifestyle.

The healthy changes, both big and small, that you have started through this challenge can develop into habits. Habits are important to develop properly because they are the foundation to consistent behavior. Habits eventually become your lifestyle autopilot, and flying though the day becomes much easier.

Questions to Consider

1. Based on today's reading, what is an action that you can take to solidify your goal setting? (See page 111 and today's action step.)

2. How has *Prescription for Life* prepared you to make healthy lifestyle choices for the rest of your life?

3. Do you know and care about someone else who would benefit from hearing about the information and strategies that you are putting into place based on *Prescription for Life* and the *Prescription for Life 21-Day Plan*?

Action Step

Your final action step is about putting it all together. Take a moment to look back at your previous action steps from Days 1–20, where you wrote down helpful information and goals.

If you would like to compile everything onto one sheet, see the following page called the *Prescription for Life 21-Day Plan— Action Steps Summary*. Place this sheet in a prominent place to review daily as your choices become habits. As your actions yield new habits, you'll experience a lifestyle that leads to a longer, healthier life!

Prescription for Life 21-Day Plan—Action Steps Summary

Day 1—From what you learned in the *Prescription for Life 21-Day Plan*, what diseases and health problems do you now know how to combat?

Day 2, 19, and 20—Record the statistics about disease prevention and living longer that motivate you most.

-
-
-
-

Day 5 and 6—List here the foods you committed to avoid in this challenge.

-
-
-

-
-
-

Day 9 and 18—Print out and continue the Personal Exercise Plan that you developed in the action steps on these days.

Day 10 and 11—Evaluate and recommit to the long-term, intermediate, and short-term goals you recorded in the action step on these days, regarding the remaining two lifestyles you can control:

Ideal weight:

-

-

-

Eating habits:

-

-

-

Day 14, 15, 16—Print out a page of the platform meals you created on these days.

Day 7, 12, 13—Record some additional helpful tips from the information presented in these days.

-

-

-

A Special Word from Dr. Richard Furman

"If I Had Only Known"

I've have shared with you my thirty years of medical experience, including my own moments of decision that made me commit to a new lifestyle. I hope *Prescription for Life* has inspired you to make a decision to live differently from now on. I became a physician because I wanted to help treat individuals who had medical problems. I look back and remember all the patients whose lives I had the privilege to improve or even save. That is the greatest reward a doctor can ever hope to receive.

But in reality, we all know that no matter what lifestyle we develop, no matter how healthy we may eat, no matter what ideal weight we chose, and no matter how strict we are with exercising, we are all someday going to pass away from this earth. Everybody is dying. From the moment you were born, you have been dying. Everything that has a beginning has an end. What then?

That is the question I made a habit of asking every cancer patient I treated in my surgical practice. I asked if they would like for me to discuss eternity with them. What happens after death? I never forced any discussion on them. I always respected our doctor-patient relationship above all else. But every single one of the patients I ever asked that question answered in the affirmative. Perhaps for the first time in their life, since they had cancer, the question of what happens after they die came to the forefront in their minds.

Pointing to the door of the examining room, I would ask, "If you were to die this moment and that were the door to heaven—and you knocked on the door—and it was opened—what could you say that would guarantee you admission?" Most answered something like, "I sure hope I've done more good than bad." One answer I will never forget came from a young man in his early thirties. He had an incurable cancer. My job was to keep him alive for as long as possible and to keep him as pain-free as I could. Knowing all the details concerning his future, it was going to be a sorrowful situation.

He was sitting on the end of the examining table with his young wife standing off to his left looking at him. His answer to the question was a story of one of the most moving, humble, and generous deeds I have ever heard (you can read the full account on pages 313–16 of *Prescription for Life*). I knew that if I held the key to heaven, I would certainly wish there was some way that deed would get him in. I told him I had never heard a better example of someone looking out for a fellow human than the story he'd just told. But I also had to explain that even as good as he and his wife had been, that encounter would not get him into heaven.

I pulled out the prescription pad from my coat pocket and wrote "John 14:6." I signed it before tearing the prescription off and handing it to him. As he took it from me and looked at the reference, I paraphrased the verse for him: "Jesus said, I am the way and the truth and the life. No man comes to the Father except by me."

And then I told him: we are all sinners, and though God does not allow any sin in heaven, he sent his Son, Jesus, to die for our sins. He died on the cross, was buried and resurrected, and is now in heaven. If we accept him as our Savior and invite him into our hearts and repent of our sins, we can be saved and admitted into heaven for eternity. I explained that if he did this, that was the answer to heaven. That is what eternity is all about.

I share this part of my medical career with you because I am interested in your health. "If I had only known" are the saddest words to hear from someone who has just been diagnosed with a severe health problem—one that could have been prevented. I want you know how to have the healthiest life possible and enjoy life to its fullest. And when the time comes that you finally think about eternity, I want you to know what I told my cancer patients. I don't want you to face the gatekeeper of heaven with the response, "If I had only known."

Your most prized possession is not your health but your soul. I want you to live younger longer—and even longer throughout eternity!

Sincerely,
Richard Furman

Medical References

Alzheimer Disease and Associated Disorders

"An Association with Great Implications: Vascular Pathology and Alzheimer Disease." 20, no. 1 (2006): 73–75.

American Heart Association

"Heart Disease and Stroke Statistics." (2004).

"Erectile Dysfunction Predicts Cardiovascular Events in High-Risk Patients." 121 (2010): 1439–46.

American Heart Journal

"Does Exercise Reduce Mortality Rates in the Elderly? Experience from the Framingham Heart Study." 128, no. 5 (1994): 965–72.

"Erectile Dysfunction: The Need to Be Evaluated, the Right to Be Treated." 150, no. 4 (2005): 620–26.

"Lifestyle Determinants of High-Density Lipoprotein Cholesterol: The National Heart, Lung, and Blood Institute Family Heart Study." 147, no. 3 (2004): 529–35.

American Journal of Cardiology

"Dietary Fiber, Lipids, and Atherosclerosis." 16 (1987): 17–22.

"Effect of Alcohol Intake and Exercise on Plasma High-Density Lipoprotein Cholesterol Subfractions and Apolipoprotein A-1 in Women." 58 (1986): 148–51.

"Efficacy of High-Intensity Exercise Training on Left Ventricular Ejection Fraction in Men with Coronary Artery Disease (the Training Level Comparison Study)." 76 (1995): 643–47.

"Management of Sexual Dysfunction in Patients with Cardiovascular Disease: Recommendations of the Princeton Consensus Panel." 86 (2000): 175–81.

"Prevention and Management of Cardiovascular Disease and Erectile Dysfunction: Toward a Common Patient-Centered Care Model." 96 (2005): 80–84.

"Usefulness of the Total Cholesterol to High-Density Lipoprotein Cholesterol Ratio in Predicting Angiographic Coronary Artery Disease in Women." 68 (1991): 1646–50.

American Journal of Clinical Nutrition

"Dietary Cholesterol from Eggs Increases the Ratio of Total Cholesterol to High-Density Lipoprotein Cholesterol in Humans: A Meta-analysis." 3 (2001): 885–91.

"Diet, Nutrition Intake, and Metabolism in Populations of High and Low Risk for Colon Cancer Relationship of Diet to Serum Lipids." 40 (1984): 921–26.

"Effects of Dietary Cholesterol on Serum Cholesterol: A Meta-analysis and Review." 55 (1992): 1060–70.

"Effects of Two Low-Fat Stanol Ester-Containing Margarines on Serum Cholesterol Concentrations as Part of a Low-Fat Diet in Hypercholesterolemic Subjects." 69 (1999): 403–10.

"Fat Preference and Adherence to a Reduced-Fat Diet." 57, no. 3 (1993): 373–81.

"High-Monounsaturated-Fat Diets for Patients with Diabetes Mellitus." 67 (1998): 577–82.

"Hypocholesterolemic Effects of Oat Bran or Bean Intake for Hypercholesterolemic Men." 40 (1984): 1146–55.

"Individual Fatty Acid Effects on Plasma Lipids and Lipoproteins: Human Studies." 65 (1997): 1628–44.

"Plasma Lipoprotein Profile and Lipolytic Activities in Response to the Substitution of Lean White Fish for Other Animal Protein Sources in Premenopausal Women." 63 (1996): 315–21.

"Plasma Lipoprotein Response to Substituting Fish for Red Meat in the Diet." 53 (1991): 1171–76.

"Red Meat Consumption and Risk of Type 2 Diabetes: Three Cohorts of United States Adults and an Updated Meta-analysis." 94 (2011): 1088–96.

"Relation of Changes in Dietary Lipids and Weight, Trial Years 1–6, to Change in Blood Lipids in the Special Intervention and Usual Care Groups in the Multiple Risk Factor Intervention Trial." 65 (1997): 272–88.

American Journal of Epidemiology

"Physical Activity as an Index of Heart Attack Risk in College Alumni." 108 (1978): 161–75.

"Prospective Study of Alcohol Consumption Quantity and Frequency and Cancer-Specific Mortality in the United States Population." 174, no. 9 (2011): 1044–53.

"Total Cholesterol and High Density Lipoprotein Cholesterol as Important Predictors of Erectile Dysfunction." 140 (1994): 930–37.

American Journal of Medicine

"Alcohol versus Exercise for Coronary Protection." 79 (1985): 231–40.

"Epidemiologic Aspects of Lipid Abnormalities." 105 (1998): 48–57.

American Journal of Surgery

"Surgery, Drugs, Lifestyle, and Hyperlipidemia." 169, no. 4 (1995): 374–78.

Annals of Epidemiology

"Lipids and Risk of Coronary Heart Disease: The Framingham Study." 2 (1992): 23–28.

Annals of Internal Medicine

"Sexual Function in Men Older Than Fifty Years of Age: Results from the Health Professionals' Follow-up Study." 139, no. 3 (2003): 161–68.

Annals of Neurology

"Dietary Fat Intake and Risk of Incident Dementia in the Rotterdam Study." 42, no. 5 (1997): 776–82.

"Dietary Fat Types and Four-Year Cognitive Change in Community-Dwelling Older Women." 72, no. 1 (2012): 124–34.

Archives of Internal Medicine

"Effect of Aerobic Exercise Training on Serum Levels of High-Density Lipoprotein Cholesterol: A Meta-analysis." 167, no. 10 (2007): 999–1008.

"The Effect of Lifestyle Modification and Cardiovascular Risk Factor Reduction on Erectile Dysfunction: A Systematic Review and Meta-analysis." 171, no. 20 (2011): 1797–1803.

"Effects of Low-Dose Niacin on High Density Lipoprotein Cholesterol and Total Cholesterol/High Density Lipoprotein Cholesterol Ratio." 148 (1988): 2493–95.

"Effects of the Amount of Exercise on Body Weight, Body Composition, and Measures of Central Obesity." 164 (2004): 31–39.

"Extended-Release Niacin vs. Gemfibrozil for the Treatment of Low Levels of High-Density Lipoprotein Cholesterol." 160, no. 8 (2000): 1177–84.

"Lifestyle for Erectile Dysfunction: A Good Choice." 172, no. 3 (2012): 295–96.

"Prescribing Exercise at Varied Levels of Intensity and Frequency: A Randomized Trial." 165, no. 20 (2005): 2362–69.

"Red Meat Consumption and Mortality. Results from Two Prospective Cohort Studies." 172, no. 7 (2012): 555–63.

"Ten-Year Follow-up of Subclinical Cardiovascular Disease and Risk of Coronary Heart Disease in the Cardiovascular Health Study." 166, no. 1 (2006): 71–78.

Archives of Neurology

"Use of Lipid-Lowering Agents, Indication Bias, and the Risk of Dementia in Community-Dwelling Elderly People." 59 (2002): 223–27.

Atherosclerosis

"Does Weight Loss Cause the Exercise-Induced Increase in Plasma High Density Lipoproteins?" 47, no. 2 (1983): 173–85.

"Relationship between Physical Activity and HDL-Cholesterol in Healthy Older Men and Women: A Cross-Sectional and Exercise Intervention Study." 127, no. 2 (1996): 177–83.

Breast Cancer Research

"Family History of Later-onset Breast Cancer, Breast Healthy Behavior and Invasive Breast Cancer among Postmenopausal Women: A Cohort Study." 12 (2010): R82.

British Journal of Cancer

"Nutrition, Lifestyle, and Colorectal Cancer Incidence: A Prospective Investigation of 10,998 Vegetarians and Non-vegetarians in the United Kingdom." 90, no. 1 (2004): 118–21.

British Medical Journal

"Alcohol and Cardiovascular Disease: The Status of the U Shaped Curve." 303 (1991): 565–68.

"Mid-life Vascular Risk Factors and Alzheimer's Disease in Later Life: Longitudinal, Population-Based Study." 322 (2001): 1447–51.

"Risk of Death from Cancer and Ischemic Heart Disease in Meat and Non-meat Eaters." 308 (1994): 1667–70.

Brown University study: *Medicine & Science in Sports & Exercise*

"Physical Activity in the Treatment of the Adulthood Overweight and Obesity: Current Evidence and Research Issues." 31 (1999): S547–52.

Canadian Journal of Cardiology

"Dietary Fiber, Complex Carbohydrate, and Coronary Artery Disease." 11 (1995): 55–62.

Chest

"Effects of Exercise Training Amount and Intensity on Peak Oxygen Consumption in Middle-Age Men and Women at Risk for Cardiovascular Disease." 128 (2005): 2788–93.

Circulation

"Aerobic Capacity in Patients Entering Cardiac Rehabilitation." 113, no. 23 (2006): 2706–12.

"Cardiovascular Implications of Erectile Dysfunction." 123, no. 21 (2011): 609–11.

"Clinical Cardiology: Physician Update: Erectile Dysfunction and Cardiovascular Disease." 123, no. 1 (2011): 98–101.

"Effect Size Estimates of Lifestyle and Dietary Changes on All-Cause Mortality in Coronary Artery Disease Patients: A Systematic Review." 112, no. 6 (2005): 924–34.

"Exercise Prescription and Proscription for Patients with Coronary Artery Disease." 112, no. 15 (2005): 2354–63.

"Impact of Cardiac Rehabilitation on Mortality and Cardiovascular Events after Percutaneous Coronary Intervention in the Community." 123, no. 21 (2011): 2344–52.

"Lipid Lowering versus Revascularization." 96, no. 4 (1997): 1360–62.

"An Overview of Randomized Trials of Rehabilitation with Exercise after Myocardial Infarction." 80, no. 2 (1989): 234–44.

"Percutaneous Coronary Intervention versus Conservative Therapy in Nonacute Coronary Artery Disease." 111, no. 22 (2005): 2906–12.

"Prevention of the Angiographic Progression of Coronary and Vein-Graft Atherosclerosis by Gemfibrozil after Coronary Bypass Surgery in Men with Low Levels of HDL Cholesterol." 96, no. 7 (1997): 2137–43.

"Red and Processed Meat Consumption and Risk of Incident Coronary Heart Disease, Stroke, and Diabetes Mellitus: A Systematic Review and Meta-analysis." 121, no. 21 (2010): 2271–83.

"Reduction of Serum Cholesterol in Postmenopausal Women with Previous Myocardial Infarction and Cholesterol Malabsorption Induced by Dietary Sitostanol Ester Margarine: Women and Dietary Sitostanol." 96, no. 12 (1997): 4226–31.

"Relationship between Erectile Dysfunction and Silent Myocardial Ischemia in Apparently Uncomplicated Type 2 Diabetic Patients." 110, no. 1 (2004): 22–26.

"Relative Intensity of Physical Activity and Risk of Coronary Heart Disease." 107, no. 8 (2003): 1110–16.

"Secondary Prevention by Raising HDL Cholesterol and Reducing Triglycerides in Patients with Coronary Artery Disease." 102, no. 1 (2000): 21–27.

"Statement on Exercise: Benefits and Recommendations for Physical Activity Programs for all Americans: A Statement for Health Professionals by the Committee on Exercise and Cardiac Rehabilitation of the Council on Clinical Cardiology, American Heart Association." 94, no. 4 (1996): 857–62.

"Third Report of the National Cholesterol Education Program. Expert Panel on Detection, Evaluation, and Treatment of High Blood Cholesterol in Adults. (Adult Treatment Panel III) Final Report." 106, no. 25 (2002): 3143–421.

Clinical Cardiology

"Brachial Artery Ultrasound: A Noninvasive Tool in the Assessment of Triglyceride-Rich Lipoproteins." 22, no. 6 Suppl. (1999): II34–39.

Diabetes Care

"Can Adoption of Regular Exercise Later in Life Prevent Metabolic Risk for Cardiovascular Disease?" 28 (2005): 694–701.

European Urology

"Association between Smoking, Passive Smoking, and Erectile Dysfunction: Results from the Boston Area Community Health Survey." 52, no. 2 (2007): 416–22.

Federal Register

"U.S. Department of Health and Human Services. Food and Drug Administration. Food Labeling; Health Claims: Soluble Fiber from Certain Foods and Coronary Heart Disease: Final Rule." 63 (1998): 8103–21.

Hypertension

"Benefit of Low-Fat over Low-Carbohydrate Diet on Endothelial Health in Obesity." 51 (2008): 376–82.

International Journal of Clinical Practice

"Endothelial Dysfunction Links Erectile Dysfunction to Heart Disease." 59, no. 2 (2005): 225–29.

"Erectile Dysfunction and Coronary Artery Disease Prediction: Evidence-Based Guidance and Consensus." 64, no. 7 (2010): 848–57.

"Past, Present, and Future: A Seven-Year Update of Sildenafil Citrate (Viagra)." 59, no. 6 (2005): 680–91.

"The Temporal Relationship between Erectile Dysfunction and Cardiovascular Disease." 61, no. 12 (2007): 2019–28.

International Journal of Impotence Research

"Dietary Factors in Erectile Dysfunction." 18, no. 4 (2006): 370–74.

"Erectile Dysfunction Association with Physical Activity Level and Physical Fitness in Men Aged 40–75 Years." 23, no. 3 (2011): 115–21.

"Erectile Dysfunction in Heart Disease Patients." 16, no. 2 (2004): 513–17.

"Mediterranean Diet Improves Erectile Function in Subjects with the Metabolic Syndrome." 18, no. 4 (2006): 405–10.

International Journal of Sports Medicine

"Comparison of Exercise and Normal Variability on HDL Cholesterol Concentrations and Lipolytic Activity." 17, no. 5 (1996): 332–37.

"Variability in the Response of HDL Cholesterol to Exercise Training in the Heritage Family Study." 23, no. 1 (2002): 1–9.

Journal of Clinical Hypertension

"Therapeutic Effect of an Interval Exercise Training Program in the Management of Erectile Dysfunction in Hypertensive Patients." 11, no. 3 (2009): 125–29.

Journal of Investigative Medicine

"Cholesterol and Coronary Heart Disease: Predicting Risks in Men by Changes in Levels and Ratios." 43 (1995): 443–50.

Journal of Nutrition

"Impact of Non-digestible Carbohydrates on Serum Lipoproteins and Risk for Cardiovascular Disease." 129 (1999): 1457–66.

"Modulation of Inflammation and Cytokine Production by Dietary Fatty Acids." 126 (1996): 1515–33.

Journal of Nutrition, Health, and Aging

"Fatty Acid Intake and the Risk of Dementia and Cognitive Decline: A Review of Clinical and Epidemiological Studies." 4, no. 4 (2000): 202–7.

Journal of Sexual Medicine

"Adherence to Mediterranean Diet and Erectile Dysfunction in Men with Type 2 Diabetes." 7, no. 5 (2010): 1911–17.

"Dietary Factors, Mediterranean Diet, and Erectile Dysfunction." 7, no. 7 (2010): 2338–45.

"Is Obesity a Further Cardiovascular Risk Factor in Patients with Erectile Dysfunction?" 7, no. 7 (2010): 2538–46.

Journal of the American Medical Association (JAMA)

"Alzheimer's Disease." 287, no. 18 (2002): 2335–38.

"Beneficial Effects of Combined Colestipol-Niacin Therapy on Coronary Atherosclerosis and Coronary Venous Bypass Grafts." 257, no. 23 (1987): 3233–40.

"Cardiac Rehabilitation after Myocardial Infarction: Combined Experience of Randomized Clinical Trials." 260, no. 7 (1988): 945–50.

"Effect of Lifestyle Changes on Erectile Dysfunction in Obese Men: A Randomized Controlled Trial." 291, no. 24 (2004): 2978–84.

"The Effects of Running Mileage and Duration on Plasma Lipoprotein Levels." 24, no. 19 (1982): 2674–79.

"Erectile Dysfunction and Subsequent Cardiovascular Disease." 294, no. 23 (2005): 2996–3002.

"Erectile Dysfunction in Obese Men." 29, no. 20 (2004): 2467.

"High-Density Lipoprotein as a Therapeutic Target: A Systematic Review." 298, no. 7 (2007): 786–98.

"The Influence of Diet on the Appearance of New Lesions in Human Coronary Arteries." 263, no. 12 (1990): 1646–52.

"Is Relationship between Serum Cholesterol and Risk of Premature Death from Coronary Heart Disease Continuous and Graded?" 256, no. 20 (1986): 2823–28.

"The Lipid Research Clinics Coronary Primary Prevention Trial Results: Reduction in Incidence of Coronary Heart Disease." 251, no. 3 (1984): 351–64.

"Meat Intake and Mortality: A Prospective Study of Over Half a Million People." 169, no. 6 (2009): 562–71.

"Multiple Risk Factor Intervention Trial." 248, no. 12 (1982): 1465–77.

"Physical Activity and Public Health. A Recommendation from the Centers for Disease Control and Prevention and the American College of Sports Medicine." 273, no. 5 (1995): 402–7.

"Physical Activity and Risk of Stroke in Women." 31 (2000): 14–18.

"Physical Activity, Diet, and Risk of Alzheimer's Disease." 302, no. 6 (2009): 627–37.

"Women Walking for Health and Fitness: How Much Is Enough?" 266, no. 23 (1991): 3295–99.

Journal of the National Cancer Institute

"Dietary Fat and Postmenopausal Invasive Breast Cancer in the National Institutes of Health-AARP Diet and Health Study Cohort." 99, no. 6 (2007): 451–62.

Journal of Urology

"Longitudinal Differences in Disease Specific Quality of Life in Men with Erectile Dysfunction: Results from the Exploratory Comprehensive Evaluation of Erectile Dysfunction Study." 169, no. 4 (2003): 1437–42.

Lancet

"Atherosclerosis Apo-lipoprotein E and the Prevalence of Dementia and Alzheimer's Disease in the Rotterdam Study." 349 (1997): 151–54.

"Convergence of Atherosclerosis and Alzheimer's Disease: Inflammation, Cholesterol, and Misfolded Proteins." 263 (2004): 1139–46.

"Effect of Potentially Modifiable Risk Factors Associated with Myocardial Infarction in Fifty-Two Countries: Case-Control Study." 364 (2004): 937–52.

"Plasma HDL Cholesterol and Risk of Myocardial Infarction: A Mendelian Randomization Study." 380 (2012): 572–80.

"Statins and the Risk of Dementia." 356 (2000): 1627–31.

Mayo Clinic Proceedings

"Erectile Dysfunction and Cardiovascular Disease: Efficacy and Safety of Phosphodiesterase Type 5 Inhibitors in Men with Both Conditions." 84, no. 2 (2009): 139–48.

"A Population-Based, Longitudinal Study of Erectile Dysfunction and Future Coronary Artery Disease." 84, no. 2 (2009): 108–13.

Metabolism

"Cholesterol Reduction by Different Plant Stanol Mixtures and with Variable Fat Intake." 48 (1999): 575–80.

"Effects of Low-Intensity Aerobic Training on the High-Density Lipoprotein Cholesterol Concentration in Healthy Elderly Subjects." 48 (1999): 984–88.

"Lipoprotein Subfractions of Runners and Sedentary Men." 35 (1986): 45–52.

"The Relationships of Vigorous Exercise, Alcohol, and Adiposity to Low and High-Density Lipoprotein-Cholesterol Levels." 53 (2004): 700–709.

National Heart, Lung, and Blood Institute (NHLBI)

"Clinical Guidelines on the Identification, Evaluation, and Treatment of Overweight and Obesity in Adults: The Evidence Report." NIH Publication No. 98-4083, September 1998.

Neurobiological Aging

"Vascular Risk Factors for Alzheimer's Disease: An Epidemiological Study." 21 (2000): 153–60.

Neuroepidemiology

"Serum Total Cholesterol, Apolipoprotein E Epsilon 4 Allele, and Alzheimer's Disease." 17 (1998): 14–20.

Neurology

"Midlife Vascular Risk Factors and Late-Life Mild Cognitive Impairment: A Population-Based Study." 56 (2001): 1683–89.

New England Journal of Medicine

"Aggressive Lipid-Lowering Therapy Compared with Angioplasty in Stable Coronary Artery Disease." 341 (1999): 70–76.

"Effects of Exercise on Plasma Lipoproteins." 348 (2003): 1494–96.

"Effects of the Amount and Intensity of Exercise on Plasma Lipoproteins." 347 (2002): 1483–92.

"Exercise to Reduce Cardiovascular Risk—How Much Is Enough?" 347 (2002): 1522–24.

"Gemfibrozil for the Secondary Prevention of Coronary Heart Disease in Men with Low Levels of High-Density Lipoprotein Cholesterol." 341 (1999): 410–18.

"Intensive versus Moderate Lipid Lowering with Statins after Acute Coronary Syndromes." 350 (2004): 1495–504.

"Light to Moderate Alcohol Consumption and the Risk of Stroke among United States Male Physicians." 341 (1999): 1557–64.

"Reduction of Serum Cholesterol with Sitostanol-Ester Margarine in a Mildly Hypercholesterolemic Population." 333 (1995): 1308–12.

"Regression of Coronary Artery Disease as a Result of Intensive Lipid-Lowering Therapy in Men with High Levels of Apolipoprotein B." 323 (1990): 1289–98.

"Silent Brain Infarcts and the Risk of Dementia and Cognitive Decline." 348 (2003): 1215–22.

"Steering Committee of the Physicians' Health Study Research Group. Final Report on the Aspirin Component of the Ongoing Physicians' Health Study." 321 (1989): 129–35.

"Trans Fatty Acids and Coronary Heart Disease." 340 (1999): 1994–98.

Nurses' Health Study: JAMA

"Moderate Alcohol Consumption during Adult Life, Drinking Patterns, and Breast Cancer Risk." 306 (2011): 1884–90.

Preventive Medicine

"Erectile Dysfunction and Coronary Risk Factors: Prospective Results from the Massachusetts Male Aging Study." 30 (2000): 328–38.

"The Multiple Risk Intervention Trial IV. Intervention of Blood Lipids." 10 (1981): 443–75.

Stroke

"Alzheimer's Disease as a Vascular Disorder: Nosological Evidence." 33, no. 4 (2002): 1152–62.

"Atherosclerosis of Cerebral Arteries in Alzheimer Disease." 35, no. 11 (2004): 2623–27.

"Exercise and Risk of Stroke in Male Physicians." 30, no. 1 (1999): 1–6.

"Leisure Time, Occupational, and Commuting Physical Activity and the Risk of Stroke." 36, no. 9 (2005): 1994–99.

"Physical Activity and Stroke Incidence: The Harvard Alumni Health Study." 29, no. 10 (1998): 2049–54.

"Physical Activity and Stroke Mortality in Women: Ten-Year Follow-up of the Nord-Trondelag Health Survey." 31, no. 1 (2000): 4–12.

"Physical Activity and Stroke Risk: A Meta-analysis." 34, no. 10 (2003): 2475–81.

"Reduction in Incident Stroke Risk with Vigorous Physical Activity: Evidence from 7.7-Year Follow-up of the National Runners' Health Study." 40, no. 5 (2009): 1921–23.

Urology

"Modifiable Risk Factors and Erectile Dysfunction: Can Lifestyle Changes Modify Risk?" 56 (2000): 302–6.

World Cancer Research Fund: Stopping Cancer Before It Starts
http://www.wcrf-uk.org/

Index

accountability, 38, 114, 311
activity, 36, 53, 92, 210, 271–72
addiction, 101–7, 124, 133, 216, 286
aerobic exercise, 229–35, 249–50
Africa, 15, 46, 117–18, 119, 281, 284
aging, 20–21, 33–34, 73
alcohol, 103, 131, 164–67, 273, 277, 282
almond milk, 153–54
alternative medicine, 76–81
Alzheimer's disease, 53–55, 122, 247–51, 259–62
American Cancer Society, 183, 267, 268, 270
American Diabetes Association, 94
American Heart Association, 74
American Institute for Cancer Research, 166, 179, 271, 273, 276
American Journal of Medicine, 165
American Stroke Association, 47
amputation, 78–79
anaerobic exercise, 237–42
anatomy, 24–25
angina, 227, 292, 294, 298, 302
Annals of Internal Medicine, 182
Annals of Neurology, 147
appearance, 185–86
appetizers, 197, 204
Archives of Internal Medicine, 86, 222, 229, 253, 305

arm muscles, 239
arteries, 19–20
    blockages of, 17, 19–20, 23, 40–43, 51–52
    and dementia, 259
    and erectile dysfunction, 292–94
    path of, 48–52
    and strokes, 43–48
aspirin, 85–87
autopilot, 108–9

back muscles, 239, 240–42
bacon, 132–33, 139, 159
"bad three" fats, 126–28
baked potatoes, 203
Benecol, 140
beta-amyloid protein, 260
beverages, 202–3
bicycling, 250
blockage, 17, 19–20, 23, 40–43, 51–52, 292–94
blood pressure, 191–92
blood sugar, 192
body fatness. *See* obesity
body mass index (BMI), 176–78, 190, 260, 305
bone density, 238
bowel movements, 151–52, 153

bowling, 250
brain
  damage of, 40, 49
  health of, 259
  vs. heart, 21
bread, 200–201
breakfast, 151–55, 281
breast cancer
  and alcohol, 166
  and exercise, 268, 271–72
  and obesity, 17
  prevention of, 119–20, 265, 276–80
Breast Cancer Research, 280
Brigham and Women's Hospital, 277
British Medical Journal, 152, 285
Brown University, 213, 251
butter, 140–41, 159

calories, 186–89, 196, 199–200, 211
cancer, 11–12
  and alternative medicine, 80–81
  as incurable, 314–15
  prevention of, 179, 265–75
candy bars, 129, 159, 211
canola oil, 140, 142, 148, 203
carotid arteries, 117
Centers for Disease Control, 95
cereal, 151–55, 248–49, 307
change, 16, 37–38, 84, 93, 150–51, 308
Cheerios, 153
cheese
  alternatives to, 156
  and artery blockage, 40
  and LDL Cholesterol, 29, 64, 72
  avoiding of, 106, 120, 137–38, 144, 159
chest pain, 227, 292, 294, 298, 302, 303
chicken, 134, 148, 156, 157, 204, 307
chips, 129–30, 159
cholesterol, 56–59, 61–65, 68–73. *See also* dietary cholesterol; High Density Lipoprotein Cholesterol; Low Density Lipoprotein Cholesterol
chronological age, 31, 37, 311
Cialis, 304
cigarettes. *See* smoking
Circulation, 292
circulatory system, 262

Coca-Cola, 202–3
coffee, 154
cognitive function, 251–52
colon cancer
  and exercise, 252, 268
  and obesity, 17
  prevention of, 119–20, 151, 281–84
  and red meat, 272, 281, 282
  and smoking, 286–87
commitment, 12, 205
  case studies in, 93–99
  to exercise, 212, 233–35
  and food, 144–45
  and goals, 109–13, 194
  and prevention, 89
  success in, 91–93
constipation, 151–52
cookies, 129, 159
core muscles, 240
couch potato, 22, 215–19, 228
crackers, 127–28
cream-based sauce, 160
crunches, 240

dancing, 250
death
  fear of, 163
  by heart disease, 191
  life after, 313–17
  as premature, 45, 86, 134, 181, 218, 245
  by stroke, 43–49, 243
decision. *See* moment of decision
dementia
  and artery blockage, 42, 50, 52–55
  and exercise, 247–52
  prevention of, 255–63
  and stroke, 40
desire, 12, 105, 132
desserts, 201
diabetes, 93–96, 161–62, 175, 306–7
Dickens, Charles, 37
diet
  around the world, 117–23
  commitment to, 12, 28–30
  and ideal weight, 173–74
  sustainability of, 147, 186
  and vegetables, 272

dietary cholesterol, 28, 54–55, 64, 67, 126–30, 136
dinner, 157–58
disability, 45, 48, 243
disease, prevention of, 243–54
dizziness, 43–44
donuts, 129, 211
Doritos, 129–30
double–blind study, 77–78
drool factor, 52–55, 248, 262

eating habits, 104
egg yolk, 135–37, 160
electrolytes, 203
emphysema, 285
endorphin, 253
erectile dysfunction, 253
    and arteries, 42
    causes of, 50–51, 291–96
    and heart disease, 297–300
    prevention of, 301–9
estrogen, 278, 279
eternity, 314–17
exercise, 12, 27–28
    as aerobic, 229–35, 249–50
    as anaerobic, 237–42
    benefits of, 209, 211–13
    and cancer, 252, 268, 283
    and cardiac output, 223–27
    and cholesterol, 71–72, 221–23
    and dementia, 247–52
    and erectile dysfunction, 307
    and losing weight, 174–75
    and medication, 88
    program for, 213–14
    and stroke, 243–47

fad diets, 29, 169, 173–74, 186–87, 200
false hope, 81
false sense of security, 85–89
fats, 67
fiber, 151–55, 196, 281, 283–84
Fiber One cereal, 153, 154
fish
    as alternative, 134, 148, 189
    and dementia, 260, 261
    and diabetes, 307

and lifestyle change, 204
and meal planning, 156, 157
and weight loss, 156
food
    around the world, 117–23
    to avoid, 131–45
    and erectile dysfunction, 306–7
    and lifestyle change, 28–30
    to live by, 146–58
    as off–limits, 159–63
Food and Drug Administration (FDA), 76–81, 165
formulas, 176–79
Framingham Heart Study, 218
fried food, 141–44, 157, 159, 187–88, 203–4
fruit
    calories of, 188
    and cancer, 272
    daily requirement of, 147–48, 151
    and dementia, 248–49
    and diabetes, 307
    and stroke prevention, 122
    and weight loss, 195–96

gardening, 250
genetics, 121
glucose, 165
goals, 109–13, 194, 311
golfing, 250
Good Samaritan, 316
grilled food, 142, 156, 157, 203
grocery shopping, 124–30

habits
    formation of, 101–9, 124
    and portions, 201–2
    returning to, 173
hamburger, 133
handball, 249–50
Harvard Medical School, 277
heart
    vs. brain, 21
    effects of weight on, 190–94
    efficiency of, 223–27
    importance of, 17, 24–25
    as muscle, 229
    strength of, 27–28

heart attack, 42, 68–69, 74, 224
heart disease, 183, 190
  and dementia, 261
  and erectile dysfunction, 297–300
heart rate, 230–32, 236, 245–46
heaven, 70, 314–17
heavy drinking, 166–67
herbal medicine, 76–81
high blood pressure, 217–18, 285
High Density Lipoprotein Cholesterol
  (HDL)
  and exercise, 87, 161, 220–23, 246
  and obesity, 183–84
  as police car, 65–67
  understanding of, 57
high fiber, 151–55
hiking, 250
horseback riding, 250
hot dogs, 133

ice cream, 138–40, 143, 159
ideal weight
  arrival at, 17, 206
  figuring of, 169, 171–80
  and food, 149
  and moment of decision, 26–27, 97
  and stroke, 47
ignorance, 135
immediate action goals, 112
inactivity. *See* sedentary lifestyle
index of oxygen demand, 225–26
inflammation, 62, 63, 222, 278
intensity, 249, 250
intermediate goals, 111–12
International Journal of Clinical Practice, 308

Japan, 121–22
jogging, 221, 229–31, 235
Journal of Clinical Oncology, 278
Journal of Nutrition, Health and Aging, 54
Journal of the American Medical Association, 166, 246–47, 248, 267, 277
Journal of Urology, 307

LaLanne, Jack, 212
leg muscles, 238–39

Levitra, 304
Lewis, C. S., 13
life expectancy
  and cholesterol, 60
  and exercise, 207–8, 232
  extending of, 21, 36
  lowering of, 182
  and jogging, 230
lifestyle, 12, 20
  change in, 84, 150–51, 269, 308
  habits of, 108
  sustainability of, 147
lipoprotein, 57
Lombardi, Vince, 99–100, 112
longevity, 210
Low Density Lipoprotein Cholesterol
  (LDL)
  and arteries, 29, 293–95
  and exercise, 246, 247
  and food, 55, 87, 137
  as lethal, 61–65
  lowering of, 71, 72, 220
  and obesity, 184
  understanding of, 57
lunch, 155–57
lung cancer, 182, 216, 265, 274, 285–87

major goals, 111
malignancy, 274
margarine, 159
Massachusetts Male Aging Study, 291–92
medical school, 21–25
medication, 83, 88, 192, 301–4
memory loss, 54
milk, 138–40, 153–54
moderation, 105, 148, 164
moment of decision
  vs. commitment, 90–91, 93–96, 100–101
  and food, 204–5
  and ideal weight, 26–27, 161–62
  and lifestyle change, 37, 144, 193–94, 313
monounsaturated fat, 67, 140, 142, 248
mortality, 13, 134, 181, 185, 226, 269
motivation to change eating habits, 112–13
muscles, 237–38

National Cancer Institute, 274
National Center for Health Statistics, 82
National Weight Control Registry, 186
Neurology, 251
New England Journal of Medicine,
    165–66
New Year's resolutions, 92
nitroglycerine, 302–3
nonfat yogurt, 154
normal weight, 176–77
Nutrition Facts box, 67, 124–30, 153
nuts, 260

oatmeal, 152, 154
obesity, 176
    and cancer, 17, 268, 282–83
    and dementia, 260
    and erectile dysfunction, 305–6
    and heart disease, 22
    penalty for, 181–84
    vs. smoking, 182–83
olive oil, 140, 142, 147, 148, 160, 203, 260
omega-3 fat, 67, 148, 157, 260
orange juice, 154
osteoporosis, 238
oxygen, 225–26

Papua New Guinea, 118–20, 281, 284
Parkinson's disease, 122
partners, 38, 311
pasta, 157, 307
pastries, 129
peer pressure, 114
penile artery, 50–51, 291–94, 302, 304–5
Penney, J. C., 100
personal testimony, 78, 80
physical activity, 210, 245, 271–72, 283
physiological age, 31, 37, 39, 98, 311
pizza, 158, 159
plaque buildup, 19–20, 39–40, 49, 64, 75,
    116, 117
platform meals, 149–58
polyunsaturated fat, 67, 140, 142
portions of food, 196–98, 201–2, 206
potassium, 203
premature mortality, 45, 86, 134, 181,
    218, 245

prevention
    of artery blockage, 51, 57–58, 69, 75
    of cancer, 265–75, 276–80, 281–84,
        285–87
    and commitment, 89
    of dementia, 255–63
    of disease, 20, 243–54
    of erectile dysfunction, 301–9
    as key to youth, 82–89
    vs. medication, 192
    need for, 91
Promise activ, 140
prostate cancer, 268, 274

quality of life, 16, 32, 210

Raisin Bran cereal, 153
red meat
    avoiding of, 30, 72, 132–35
    and colon cancer, 272, 281, 282
    and LDL Cholesterol, 64, 120
regaining weight, 173–74, 186–87
rehabilitation, 226–27
resting heart rate, 236, 245–46
rice milk, 153–54
Rotterdam Study, 260–61, 262
Rush University Medical Center (Chi-
    cago), 110

salad, 155–56, 157, 197, 204, 307
salmon, 134, 136, 189, 197
sandwich, 156
saturated fat
    avoiding of, 126–30, 132
    and dementia, 54–55
    as harmful, 28–30, 67, 106
    and LDL Cholesterol, 64
sausage, 159
scar tissue, 62–63
sedentary lifestyle, 210, 215–19, 268
self-control, 102
shame, 171, 205
shoulder muscles, 239
side effects, 87–88
silent strokes, 262
sin, 316
skim milk, 138, 153–54, 159

smoking
    and addiction, 101–5, 107
    and lifestyle change, 131
    and lung cancer, 265, 274, 285–87
    vs. obesity, 182–83
    and sedentary lifestyle, 216–17
smoothie, 147, 154, 173
snacks, 198–99, 200, 206, 210–11
sodium, 84, 203
soup, 156, 157, 197, 204
soy milk, 153–54
splinter syndrome, 62–64
steak, 30, 132–35
strength, 237
stroke, 40, 42–48, 162, 183, 243–47
stupidity, 135
sugar, 200–201, 203, 295
swimming, 250

ten-minute factor, 101–7
tennis, 22, 116, 250, 251
testosterone, 289, 291, 295–96
third world, 117–20
thirty-minute exercise program, 232–35
Total Cholesterol, 59–61, 66–67, 71, 72
trans fat, 64, 67, 106, 126–30
transient ischemic attack (TIA), 45, 47
triglycerides, 59
tuna, 136, 189, 197

University of North Carolina at Chapel
    Hill, 271
Urology, 253

vascular dementia, 54, 247–48, 259–62
vegetables
    and Alzheimer's disease, 248–49
    and cancer, 272
    daily requirement of, 147–48, 151
    and diabetes, 307
    calories of, 155, 188
    and weight loss, 195–96
Viagra, 304
victory, 112–13

walking, 218, 231, 233–35, 250
warning signs, 56–59, 74–75, 299–300,
    309
weight
    controlling of, 199–204
    effect on heart, 190–94
    loss of, 195–99, 277–80
    maintaining of, 270–71
    regaining of, 173–74, 186–87
weight lifting, 239
Weight Watchers, 155, 188
whole grain, 148, 152, 200, 307
whole milk, 138–40, 159
wine, 164, 273, 277
World Cancer Research Fund, 166, 179,
    270–71, 273

Richard Furman, MD, FACS, spent over thirty years as a vascular surgeon. He is passionate about helping people prevent the problem that kills over half of all Americans. Furman is past president of the North Carolina Chapter of the American College of Surgeons, past president of the North Carolina Surgical Society, and a two-term governor of the American College of Surgeons. He is cofounder of World Medical Mission, the medical arm of Samaritan's Purse, and is a member of the board of Samaritan's Purse. He lives in North Carolina.

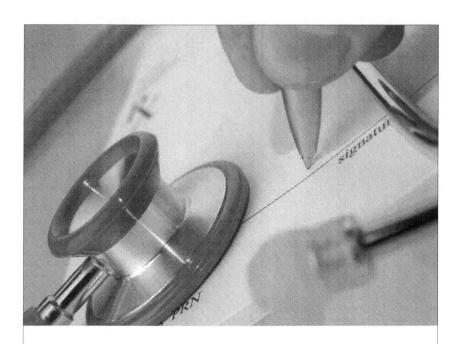

Visit
PRESCRIPTIONFORLIFEPLAN.COM
to Read Dr. Furman's Blog
and Stay Connected

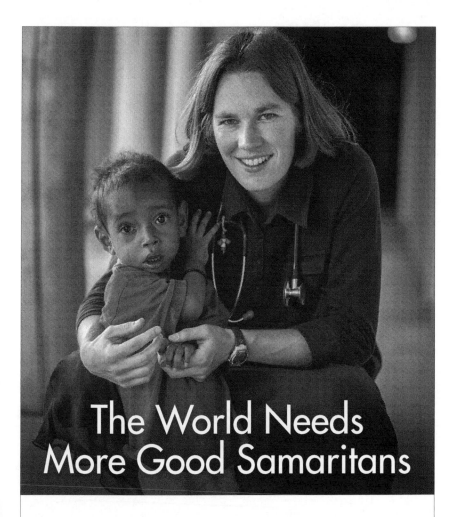
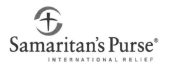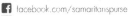

Bestselling author **Linda Evans Shepherd** helps women tap into the deeper resources of God so they can discover how to tame their stress, still their fears, and calm their hearts.

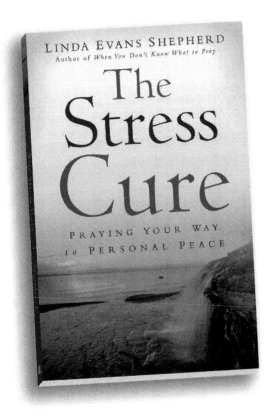

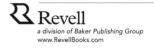

Revell
a division of Baker Publishing Group
www.RevellBooks.com

Available wherever books and ebooks are sold.

"Anti-Fat Pastor" **Steve Reynolds** reveals four keys that lead to health and fitness. He shares the simple lifestyle changes—both inside and out—that led to his own incredible weight loss, and he invites you to change your life forever by committing your body to God.

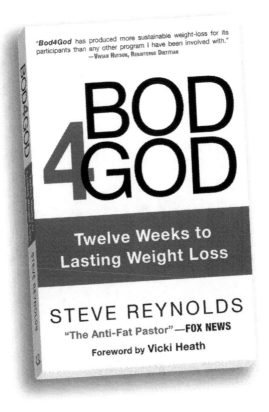

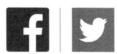